Romantic Massage

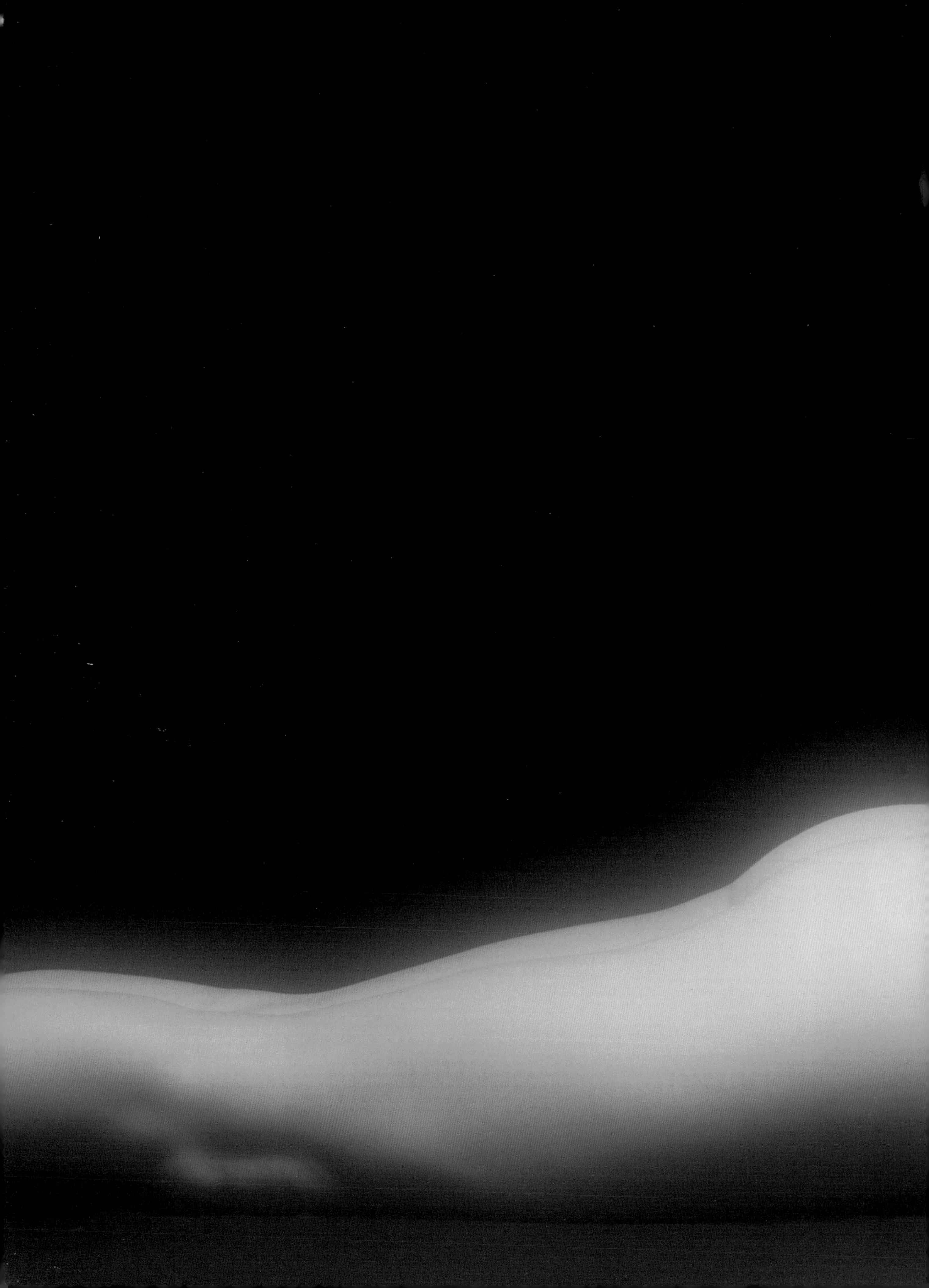

Romantic Massage

RJ Nikola, LMT

Sterling Publishing Co., Inc., New York
A Sterling/Chapelle Book

Chapelle Ltd.

Owner: Jo Packham

Editor: Linda Orton

Staff: Marie Barber, Malissa Boatwright, Kass Burchett, Rebecca Christensen, Michael Hannah, Holly Hollingsworth, Pauline Locke, Ginger Mikkelsen, Karmen Quinney, Leslie Ridenour, and Cindy Stoeckl

Photography: Ryne Hazen and Kevin Dilley for Hazen Photography, Ogden, Utah

Photo Stylist: Cheri Herrick, Jo Packham

Hair Stylist: Becky Porter, Cheri Teuscher

Make-up Artist: Holly Browning

Models: Jennifer Emperador, Suzi Ivie, Frank Slaugh, Ryanne Webster, Jason Williams, Dave Yei

A special thank you to Scott and Kelly Buehler, Ogden, Utah, for allowing us to photograph part of this book in their home, also, to The Alaskan Inn, Ogden, Utah, where some of the photographs in Chapter 6 were taken. Their trust and cooperation is greatly appreciated.

Library of Congress Cataloging-in-Publication Data

Nikola, R. J.
Romantic Massage / R.J. Nikola
p. cm.
"A Sterling/Chapelle Book"
Includes index.
ISBN 0-8069-9973-X
1. Massage. 2. Sexual Exitement. 3. Intimacy (Psychology)
I. Title.
RA780.5.N55 1997
613.9'6--dc21 97-21597
CIP

10 9 8 7 6 5 4 3 2 1

Published by Sterling Publishing Company, Inc.
387 Park Avenue South, New York, NY 10016

Distributed in Canada by Sterling Publishing
c/o Canadian Manda Group, One Atlantic Avenue, Suite 105
Toronto, Ontario, Canada M6K 3E7
Distributed in Great Britain and Europe by Cassell PLC
Wellington House, 125 Strand, London WC2R 0BB, England
Distributed in Australia by Capricorn Link (Australia) Pty Ltd.
P.O. Box 6651, Baulkham Hills, Business Centre, NSW 2153, Australia
Printed in Hong Kong

Sterling ISBN 0-8069-9973-X

Every effort has been made to ensure that all of the information in this book is accurate. However, due to differing conditions and individual skills, the publisher cannot be responsible for any injuries, losses, and/or other damages which may result from the use of the information in this book.

If you have any questions or comments please contact:

Chapelle Ltd., Inc.
P.O. Box 9252
Ogden, UT 84409

Phone: (801) 621-2777
FAX: (801) 621-2788

preface

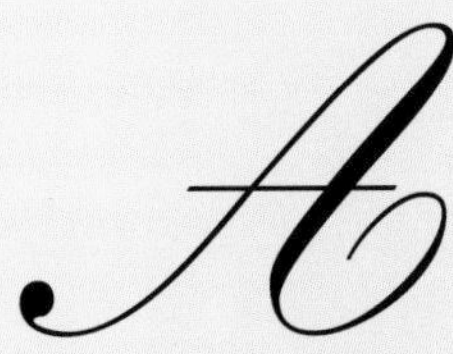

As a licensed massage therapist, I have had the opportunity to meet people who come into my office celebrating a birthday, an anniversary, or other special occasion wanting a massage or spa service for their spouses. Sometimes both desire a massage. But more often, it is only one partner that receives massage. While purchasing a massage is a selfless gift and token of their affection, it is unfortunate that both lovers cannot enjoy massage from one another's hands. It not only soothes sore muscles and calms tired minds, it is a beautiful expression of tenderness. A therapist's hand may be more skilled, but only a lover's touch can express love, passion, and sensuality.

I remember when I was studying massage and wanted to practice on my wife. Once she began to receive massage from me on a regular basis, she realized the benefits; not only to her health, but to our relationship as well.

From the very beginning, I had, as it were, a revelation. I discovered all the subtle variations of my partner's body; the tight muscles that held her stress, the stiffness that needed to be stretched out, the tender parts wanting to be gentled. I had overlooked these before. I then began to understand the little aches and pains she silently endured on a daily basis.

I seemed to constantly complain about my back pain or my sore feet. My wife never once said, "I ache too." I found myself touching her not for intimacy alone, but to bring relief to her sore shoulders, to ease the pain in her lower back and hips or tired feet from standing long hours. I developed a sensitivity to her needs and desired to help her feel better.

In the process, she noticed my concern and love. Massage deepened our feelings for each other. It awakened within us those emotions that tend to fall to the side in relationships as people grow accustomed to each other. We grew closer because of this heightened awareness.

I write this book for couples and lovers who want to learn through massage how to rekindle something romantic, something tender, something intimate in themselves and each other.

RJ Nikola, LMT
Director of
Europa Therapeutic Massage & Acupressure Clinic

About the Author

RJ Nikola is a licensed massage therapist and the author of several health-related books used in massage therapy schools throughout the United States. He is an instructor of massage, shiatsu, and hydrotherapy.

Mr. Nikola has a successful practice in the mountainwest region of the U.S., where he is director of a European style day spa and massage clinic.

He received his formal schooling in somatic therapies in North America. He has received additional training in massage and acupressure in western and eastern Europe.

Mr. Nikola has shared his knowledge and skills with others by teaching and writing. He has traveled to Europe on several occasions to do research on spa techniques and healing modalities at world class health centers.

Table of Contents

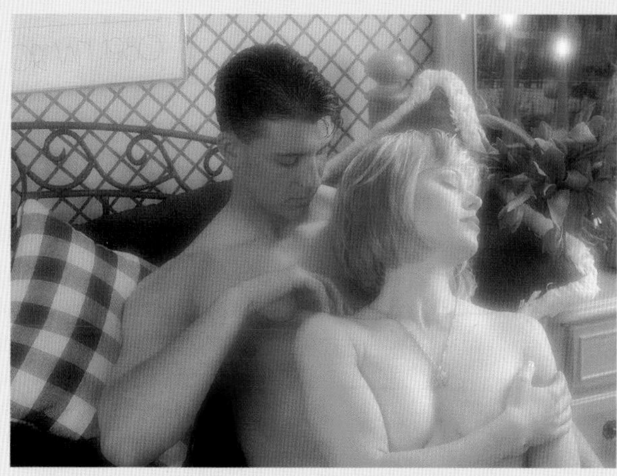

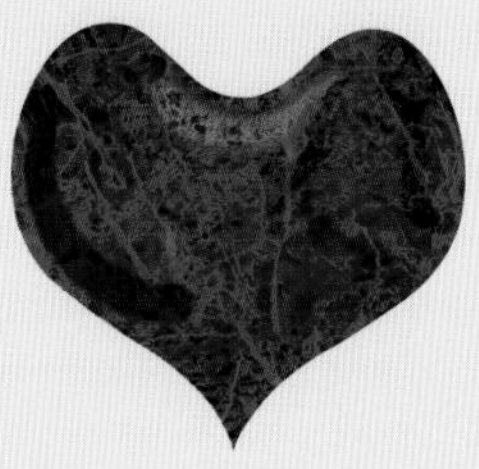

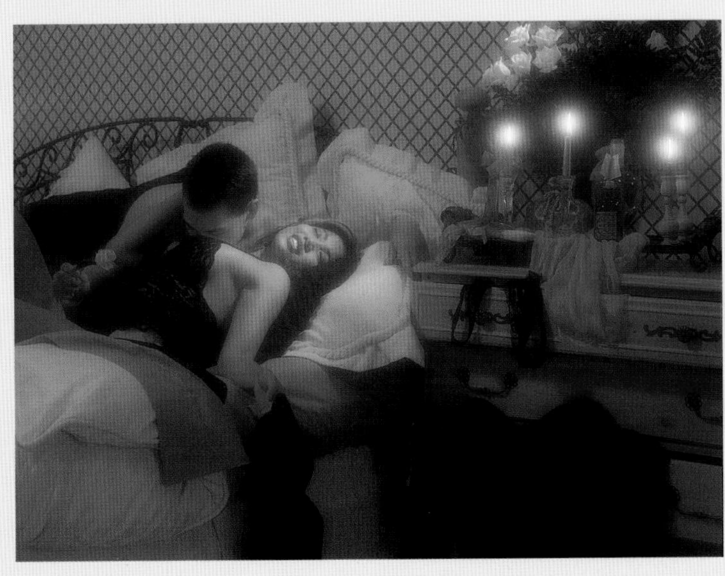

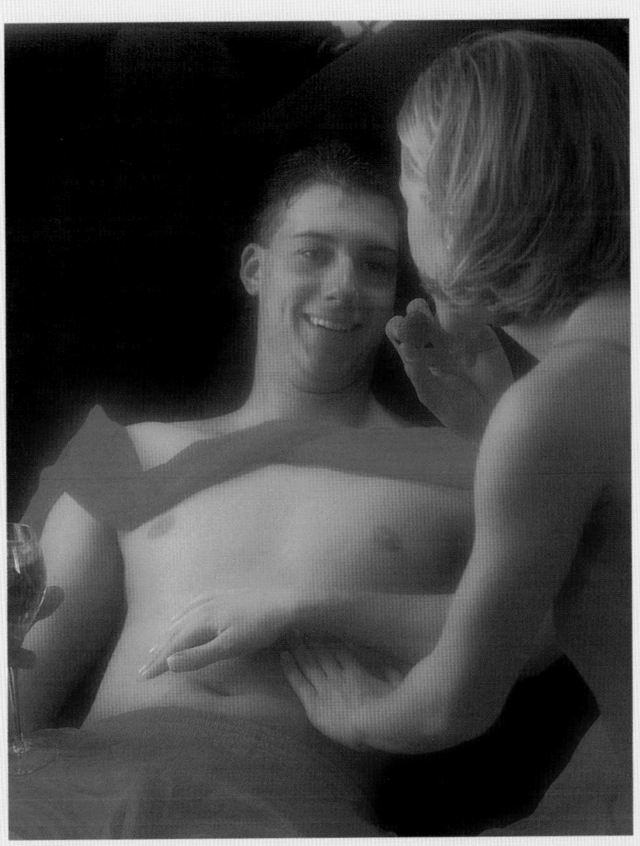

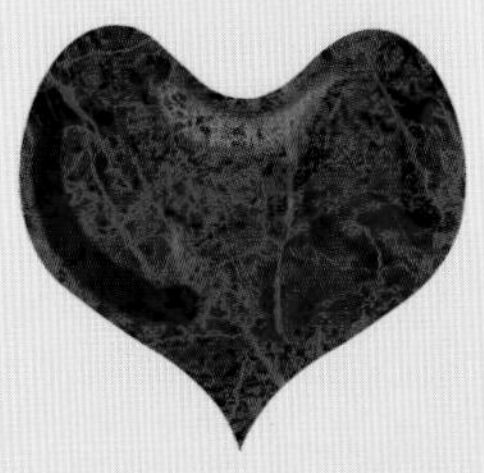

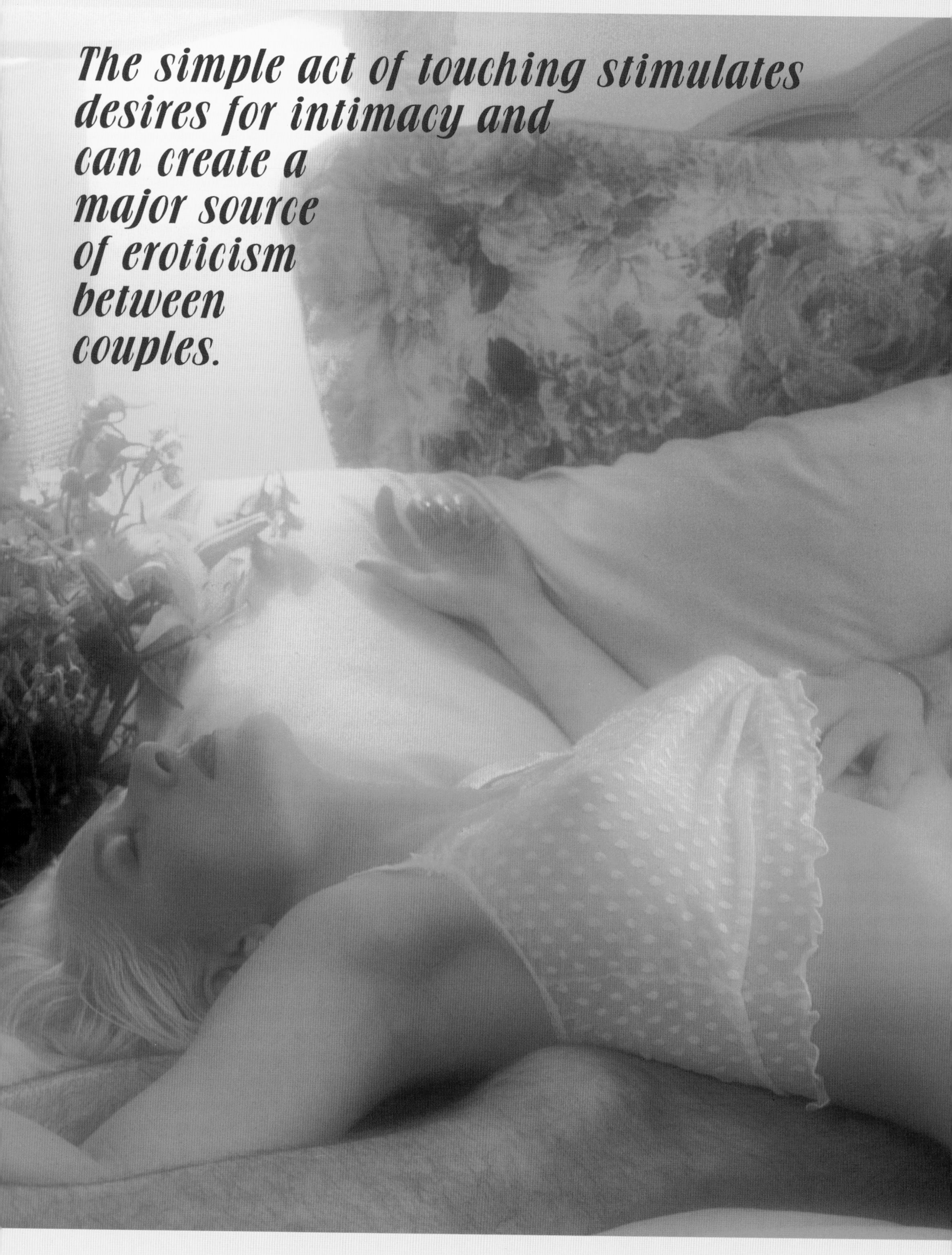
The simple act of touching stimulates
desires for intimacy and
can create a
major source
of eroticism
between
couples.

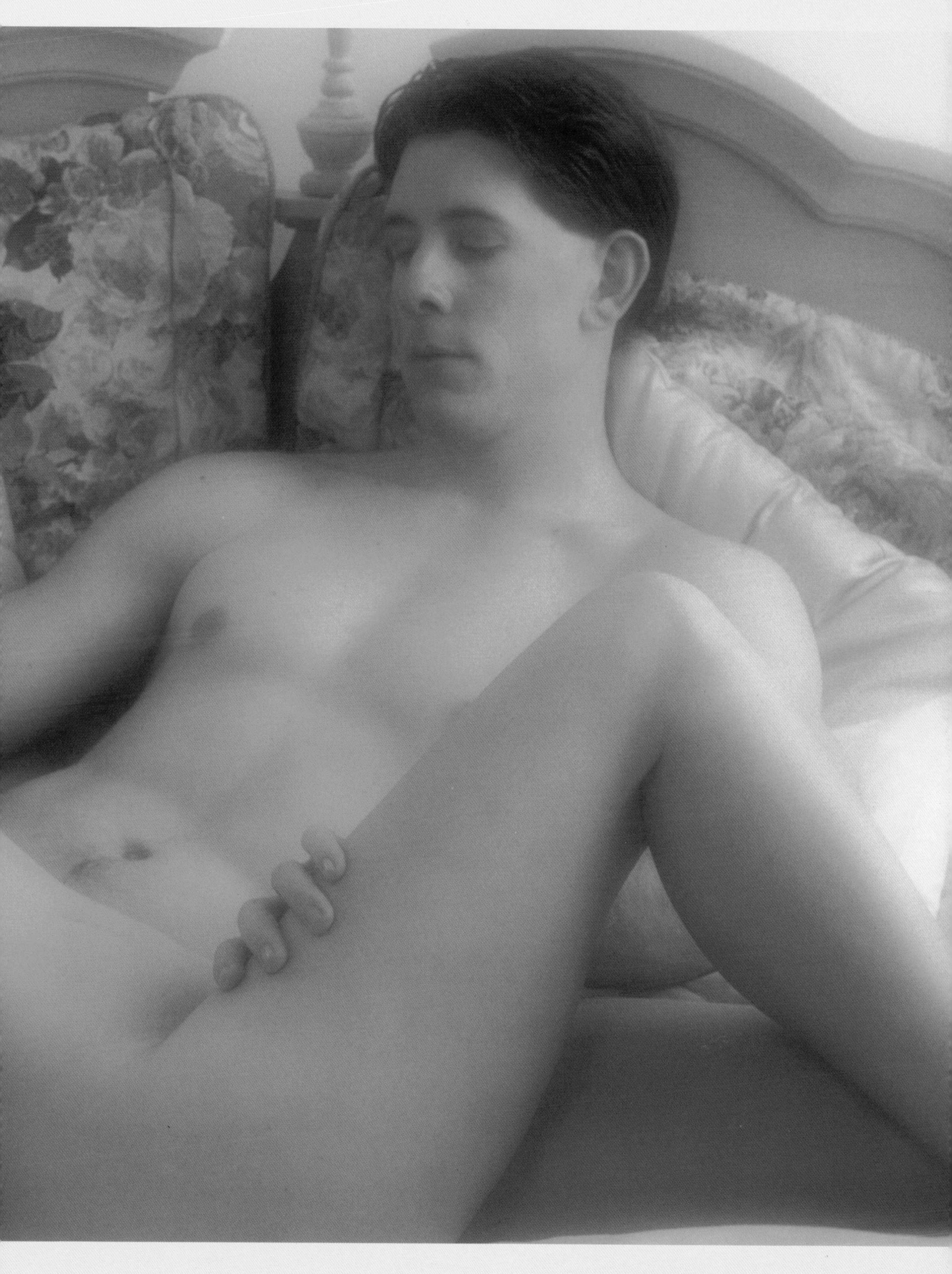

chapter one

Language of Touch

Touch is, by far, the most important of the senses and the first to develop in the human embryo. Of all the senses, touch involves the entire body. The wondrous thing about touch is that it not only involves sensory input — as do all the senses — it also conveys information: the hearty handshake of friendly neighbors, a congratulatory pat on the back, the tender embrace of a loved one, or a lingering kiss that discloses intimate feelings.

This powerful ability to share and receive information through touch is as old as human history itself.

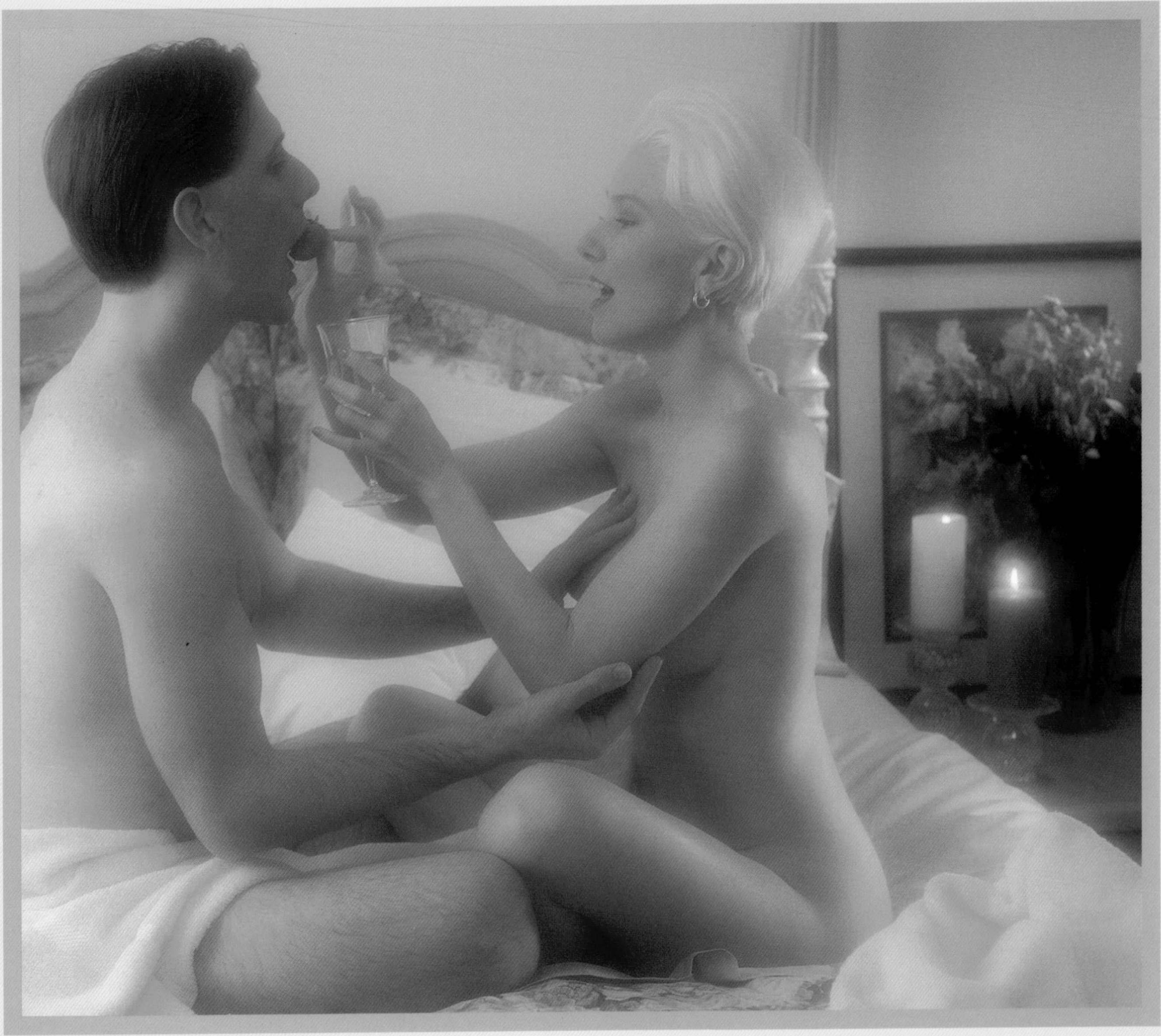

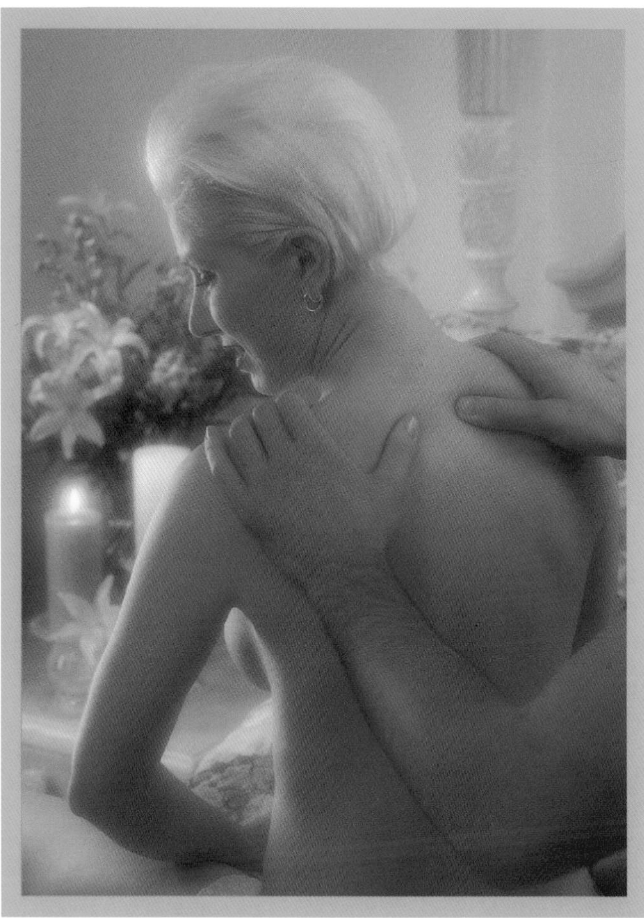

Massage can be used to promote relaxation, health, and healing. Rubbing out sore, stiff shoulder muscles will help your partner to relax.

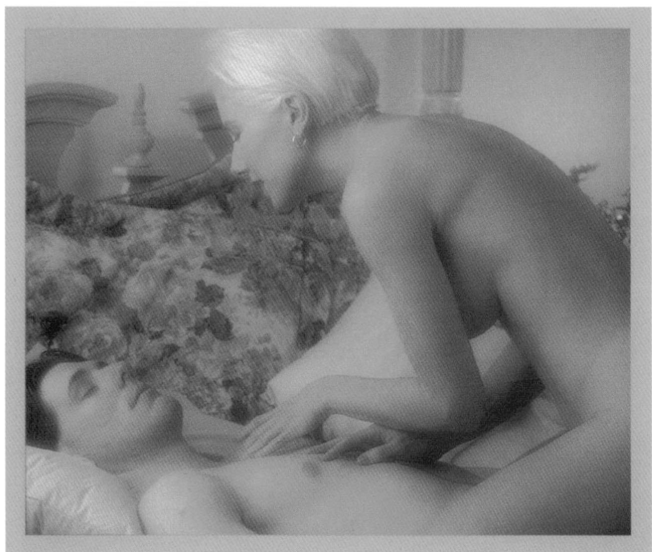

Massage can also be used to convey feelings of love and intimacy to one's partner. Sexual desire may be stirred through close contact and light touch.

The History of Massage

Touch for healing purposes (massage) has a rich heritage that dates back many thousands of years. As far back as 3000 B.C., the people of China were using massage, acupuncture, and herbal remedies as their healing system. Approximately 1800 B.C., the Ayurveda of India recommended rubbing and shampooing the skin to assist the body's self-healing powers. The Greek physician Hippocrates, known as the "Father of Medicine", regularly incorporated massage, hydrotherapy (using water to heal), and herbs for treatment of patients' illnesses. Romans used massage as an integral part of their approach to holistic health.

Massage continued to be an important part of health and healing until the middle ages when massage began to fall into disrepute because of strict religious doctrines. Christian religious leaders felt that massage invoked the sensual pleasures of the flesh. Consequently, bath houses were closed and massage was no longer practiced.

With the Renaissance came renewed interest and appreciation for the human form. Physicians began to explore the body within and without. Leonardo da Vinci compiled large volumes of anatomical sketches that showed the structure of the body along with theories on how it functioned. Royalty saw the wisdom in this approach as opposed to blood letting with leaches and needles, or cauterizing with red hot knives. Soon it became fashionable for the wealthy to have a personal physician and masseuse or masseur.

In the nineteenth century Dr. Henrik Ling brought the massage skills of China to Sweden for gymnastic athletes. This was the beginning of what we refer to as "Swedish" massage.

> *"Men are motivated and empowered when they feel needed...*
> *Women are motivated and empowered when they feel cherished."*
>
> *John Gray, Ph.D.*

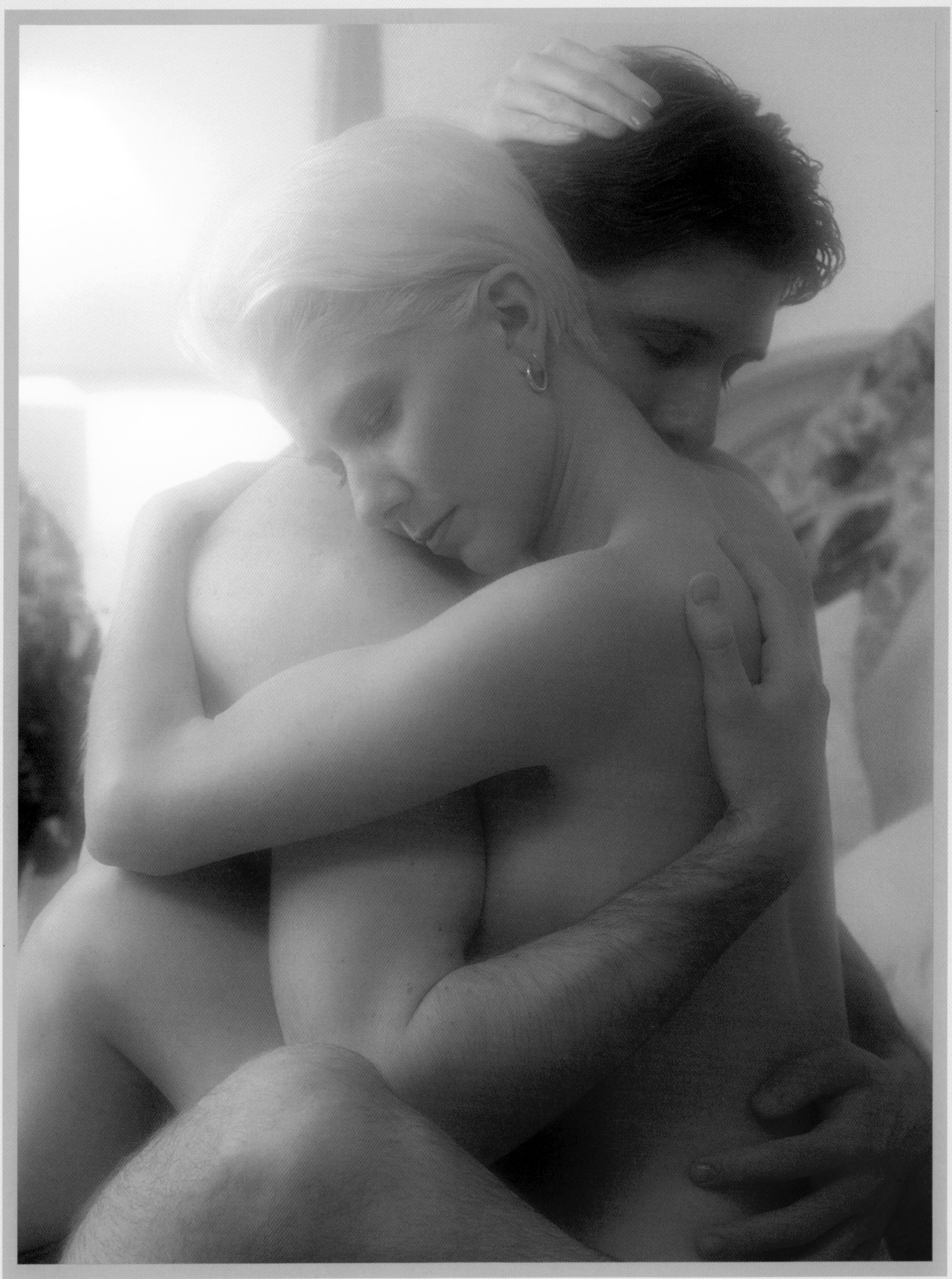

Personal Relationships

"Swedish" massage may have originally been associated with athletic or medicinal purposes, but, because of the sense of touch, it also can be used for romantic purposes. If you want to have a therapeutic massage, you may go to a massage therapist, chiropractor, or physical therapist. However, if the purpose is pleasure, massage can be experienced best when shared by loving partners. It arouses the senses. It stimulates interests. It relaxes inhibitions. Massage stimulates desires for intimacy. The simple act of touching can do this and more. Massage can be an important part — better yet, an essential part — of an intimate sexual relationship between couples. It intensifies feelings.

What makes a massage so magical, behind closed doors or in a secluded setting, is the innocent childlike freedom to touch and explore. A flood of pleasurable sensations allows feelings to unfold gracefully and naturally without agendas, timelines, or reminders of the world outside the bedroom door. It can be a beautiful extension of love, a prelude of things to come, an enhancement of lovemaking, and a prolonging of intimacy.

Did you Know?
February is Creative Romance Month.
March is Poetry Month.
June is National Rose Month.
August is Romance Awareness Month.
August 25th is Kiss and Make-Up Day

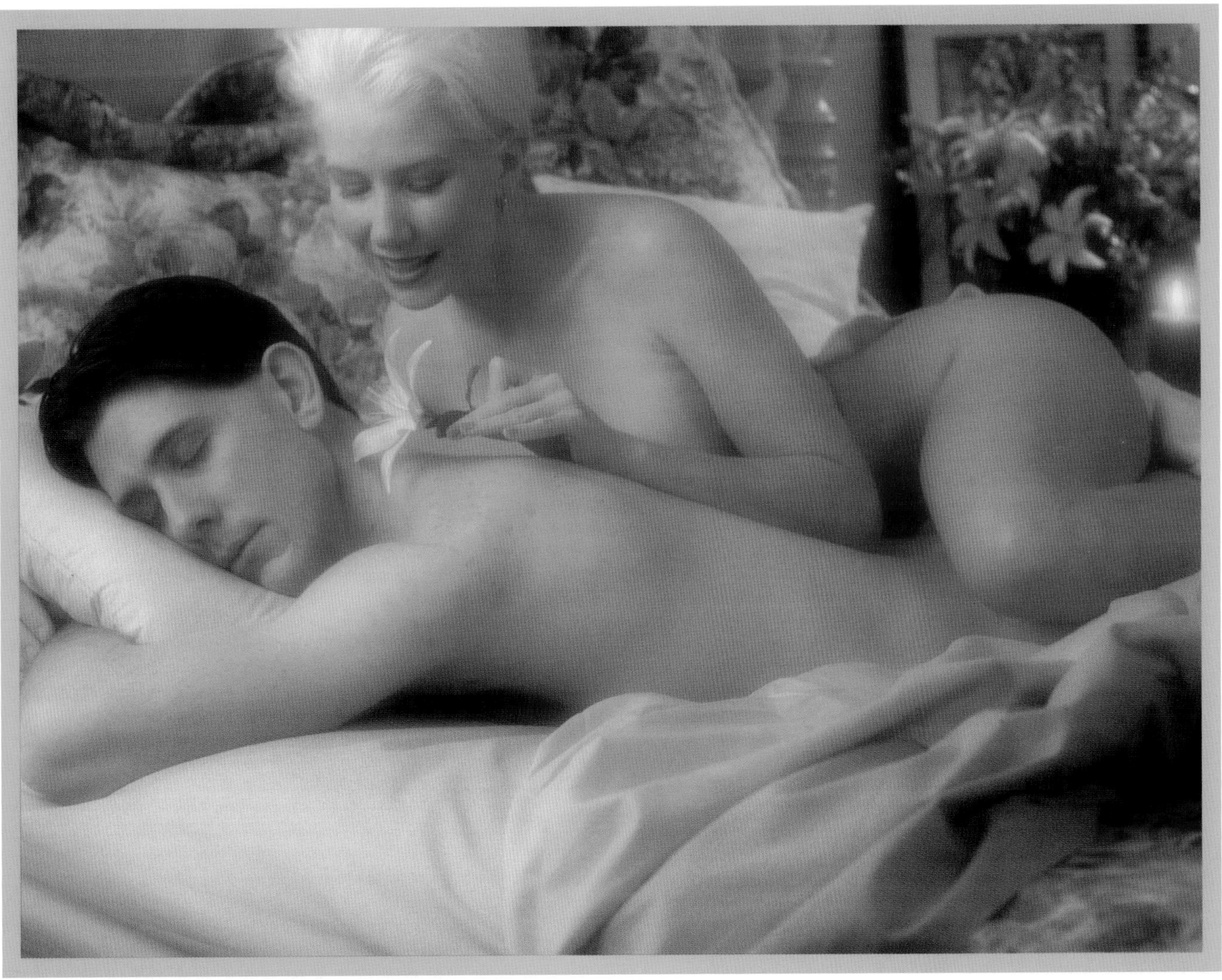

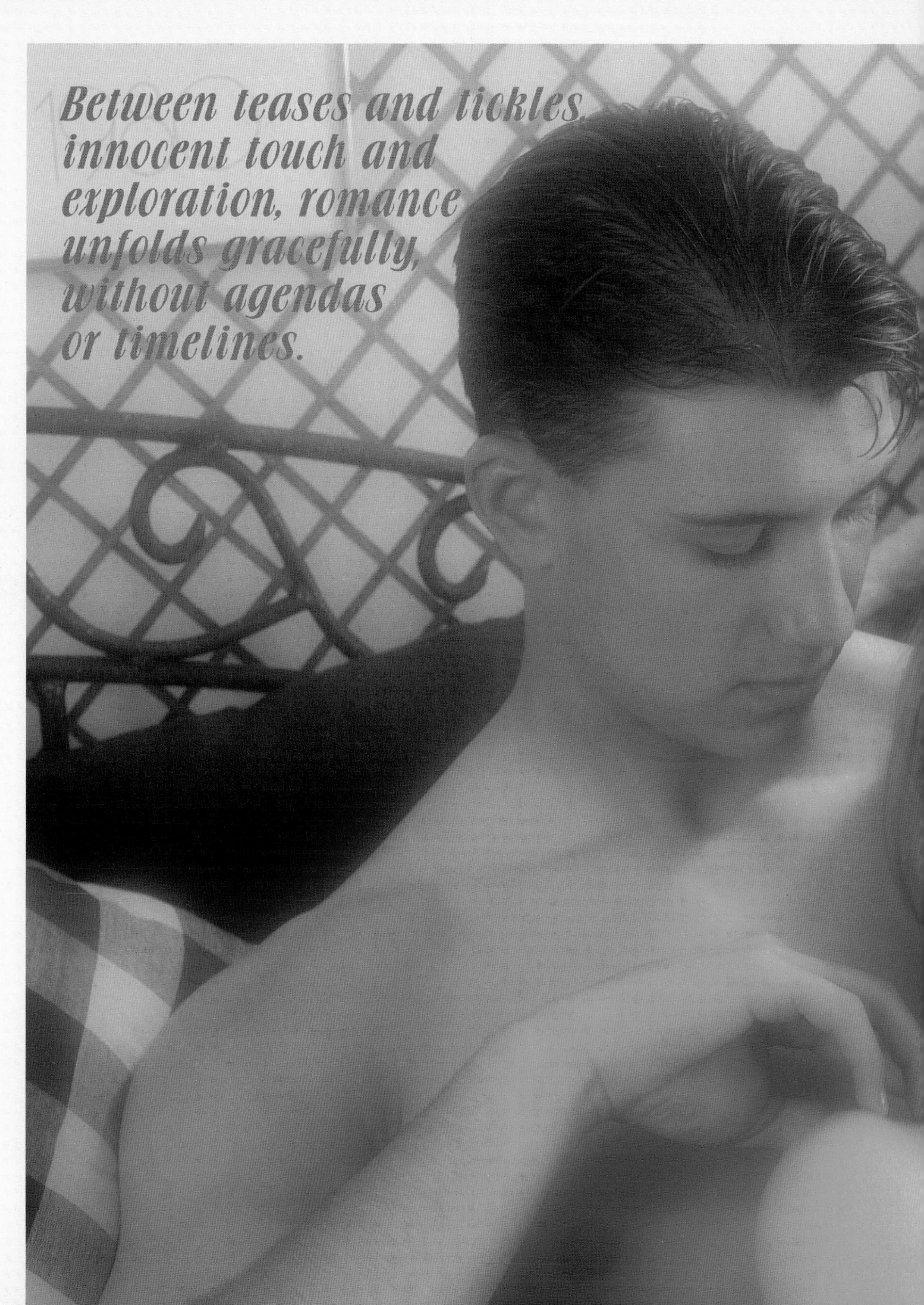
Between teases and tickles,
innocent touch and
exploration, romance
unfolds gracefully,
without agendas
or timelines.

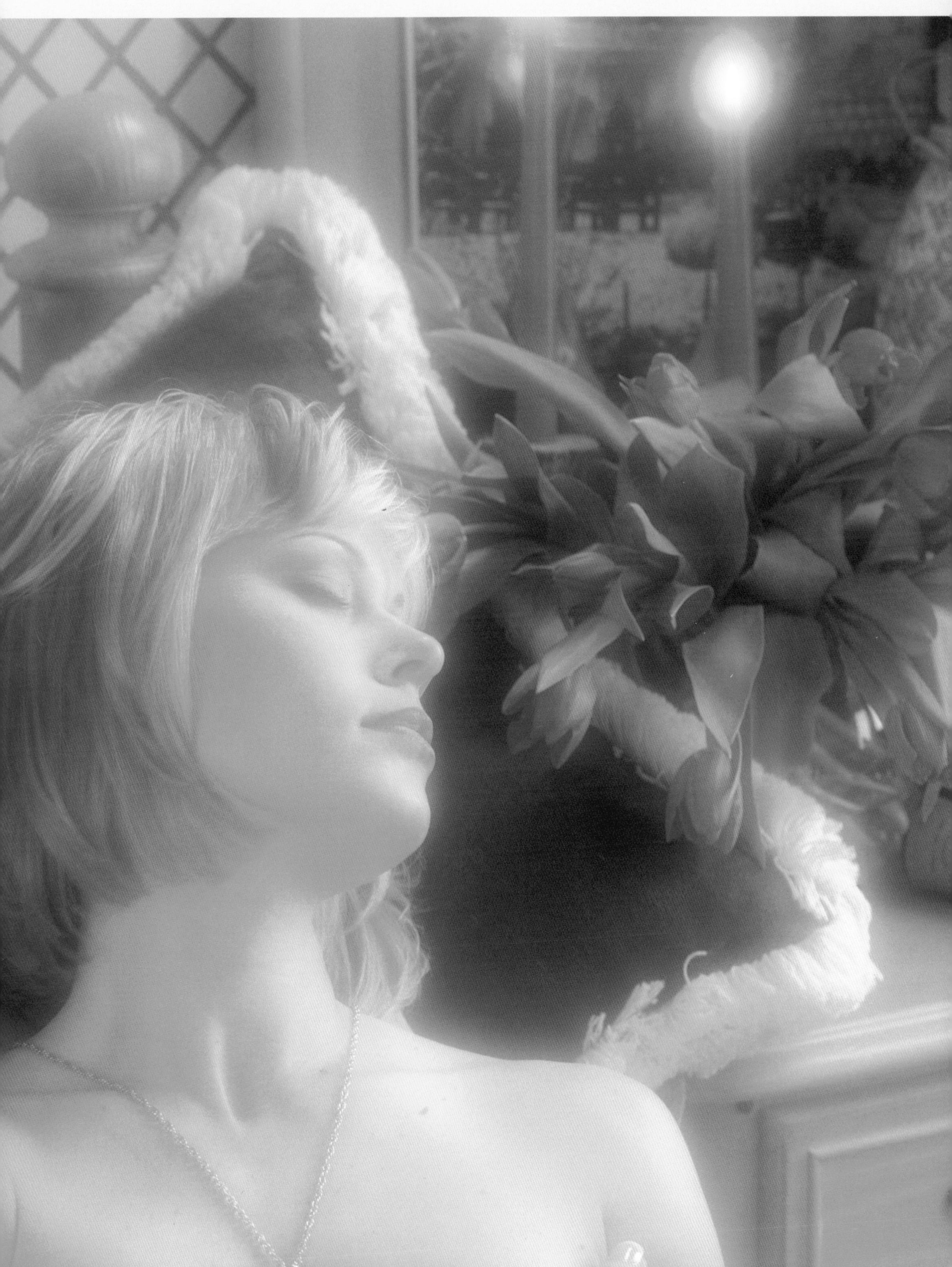

chapter two

Skin & Sensitivity

Our skin is the largest organ in the human body. It is not only an organ of respiration — it breathes — it is an enormously complex touch receptor that floods our minds with information. Through skin we receive information about an object. Is it hot or cold, hard or soft, dry or damp , smooth or rough, sharp or dull?

All of this incoming information from our skin allows us to perceive our immediate world, form opinions of it, and shape the realities of our lives around it.

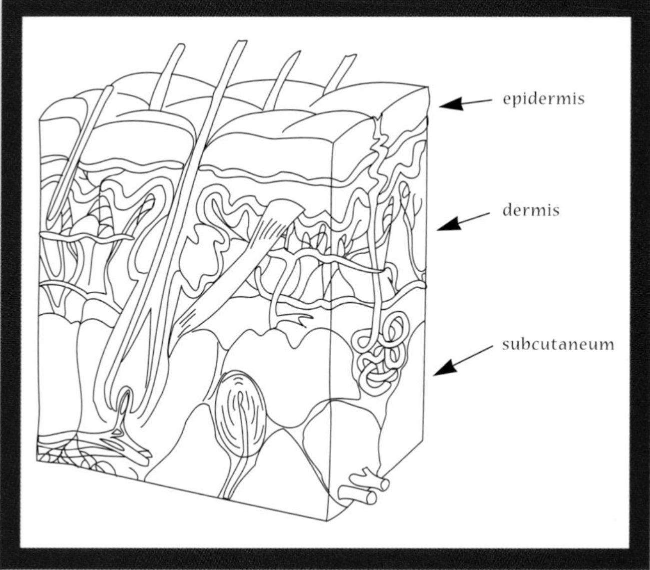

Physiology of the Skin

The skin has three basic layers of tissues:

- **epidermis**
- **dermis**
- **subcutaneum**

The **epidermis**, approximately as thick as a sheet of paper, protects deeper layers of skin from damage and dehydration. It can become dry, chaffed, and needs moisture for replenishment. That is why bathing with oils and massage keep skin soft and supple.

The **dermis**, the second layer, has blood vessels that feed the skin, nerves, hair follicles, and glands. Thickness varies from five to twenty-five times the thickness of the epidermis. It is thinnest on the eyelids and thickest on the bottom of the feet.

The deepest layer, the **subcutaneum**, is composed of fatty tissue that helps glue the top layers of skin to the muscle and bone beneath. This last layer of skin, contains larger blood vessels, nerves, and the base of hair follicles.

Flower of the Month

January	*Carnation*
February	*Violets*
March	*Jonquil*
April	*Sweet pea*
May	*Lily of the valley*
June	*Rose*
July	*Larkspur*
August	*Gladiolus*
September	*Aster*
October	*Calendula*
November	*Chrysanthemum*
December	*Narcissus*

Surprise your lover with a "Flower of the Month"

Nerve Receptors

There are over half a million nerve receptors in the body that act as sentinels to alert us of any sensation. Some sensations warn us of danger, others announce long awaited pleasures. The heaviest concentrations of nerve endings occur on the lips and fingers, the least concentrated are along the back. Usually, the more erogenous the zone, the more nerve endings it contains.

Some receptors, located just beneath the surface of the skin, are highly sensitive to the slightest touch. Others sense deeper pressures and vibrations. Some record the movement of each and every hair on the body. Still others inform us of temperature variations as well as pleasures and pains. Nerves help us explore the world around us and massage helps these nerves achieve and maintain a state of health and happiness.

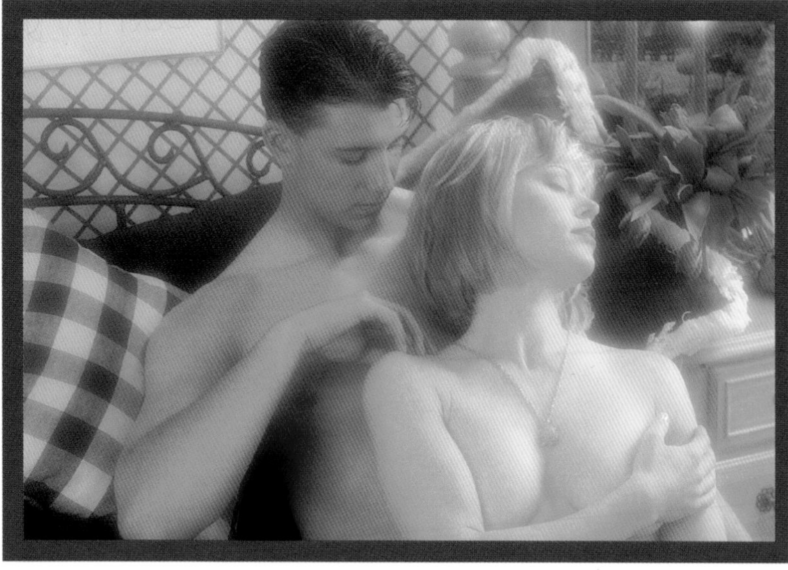

"Meissner's corpuscles" are acutely sensitive to very light touch. They are located just beneath the surface of the skin and track movement with precision.

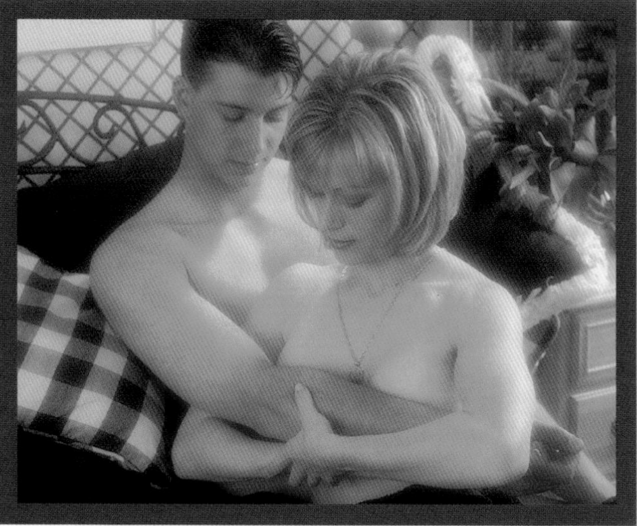

"Pacinian corpuscles" are located further below the skin's surface. They sense both deep pressures and vibrations.

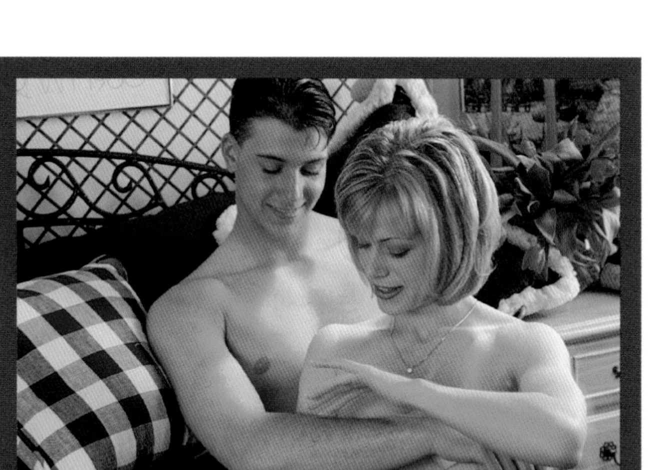

"Hair end organs" are delicate nerve endings that wrap around the base of each hair follicle. Whenever a hair is brushed, this nerve records the slightest movement.

> *"A good lover is like a gourmet. He or she takes the time to seduce not only the body but also the heart and soul. This allows for sexual energy to build up slowly. And the longer you allow sexual energy to circulate in your body, the more powerful its effects."*
>
> *Barbara De Angelis, Ph.D.*

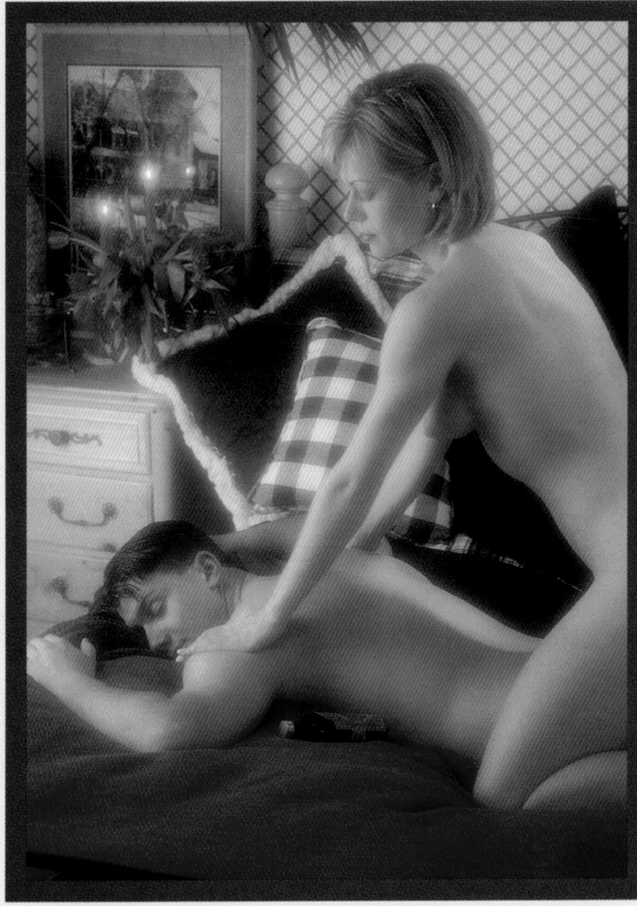

Benefits of Massage

The benefits of massage are many and far reaching. They affect the body, the mind, and the spirit.

The physical benefits of massage are:

- ♥ Deep relaxation and stress reduction
- ♥ Relief of muscular tension/stiffness
- ♥ Reduced muscle spasm and pain
- ♥ Greater joint flexibility and increased range of motion
- ♥ Promotion of deeper, easier breathing
- ♥ Better circulation of blood and lymph fluids
- ♥ Reduction of high blood pressure
- ♥ Relief of tension headaches and eyestrain
- ♥ Healthier, better nourished skin
- ♥ Quicker recovery from pulled muscles and sprained ligaments

The mental/emotional benefits of massage are:

- ♥ Relaxed and focused state of alertness
- ♥ Reduced mental stress and calm mind
- ♥ Increased ability to adapt to stressors
- ♥ Greater capacity for clearer thinking
- ♥ Satisfied need for nurturing touch
- ♥ Feelings of general well-being
- ♥ Reduced anxiety and depression
- ♥ Greater awareness of body/mind connection

The sensual/sexual benefits of massage are:

- ♥ Increased body awareness to sensations
- ♥ Heightened sensitivity to erogenous zones
- ♥ Appreciated response to a partner's touch
- ♥ Ease of relaxation and release of inhibitions
- ♥ Healthy and pleasurable form of foreplay
- ♥ Natural expression of love

Contraindications to Massage

The contraindications to romantic massage are a list of common sense precautions for the health of both your partner and yourself.

Do not give a massage if:

- ♥ Either partner has a FEVER. Fever is the body's way of fighting disease.
- ♥ Either partner has an OPEN WOUND. Depending on the size of the wound, proceed with caution.
- ♥ Either partner has a SKIN INFECTION. Massage may aggravate the condition or spread the infection to adjoining areas or to the other person.
- ♥ Either partner has a serious HEART PROBLEM or a BLOOD CLOTTING condition. Massage could make matters worse.
- ♥ Either partner is ILL.
- ♥ Either partner has had a SURGICAL PROCEDURE using a general anesthesia in the previous 6 to 8 weeks.
- ♥ If there is any question about massage, consult a professional *massage therapist* or *physician*.

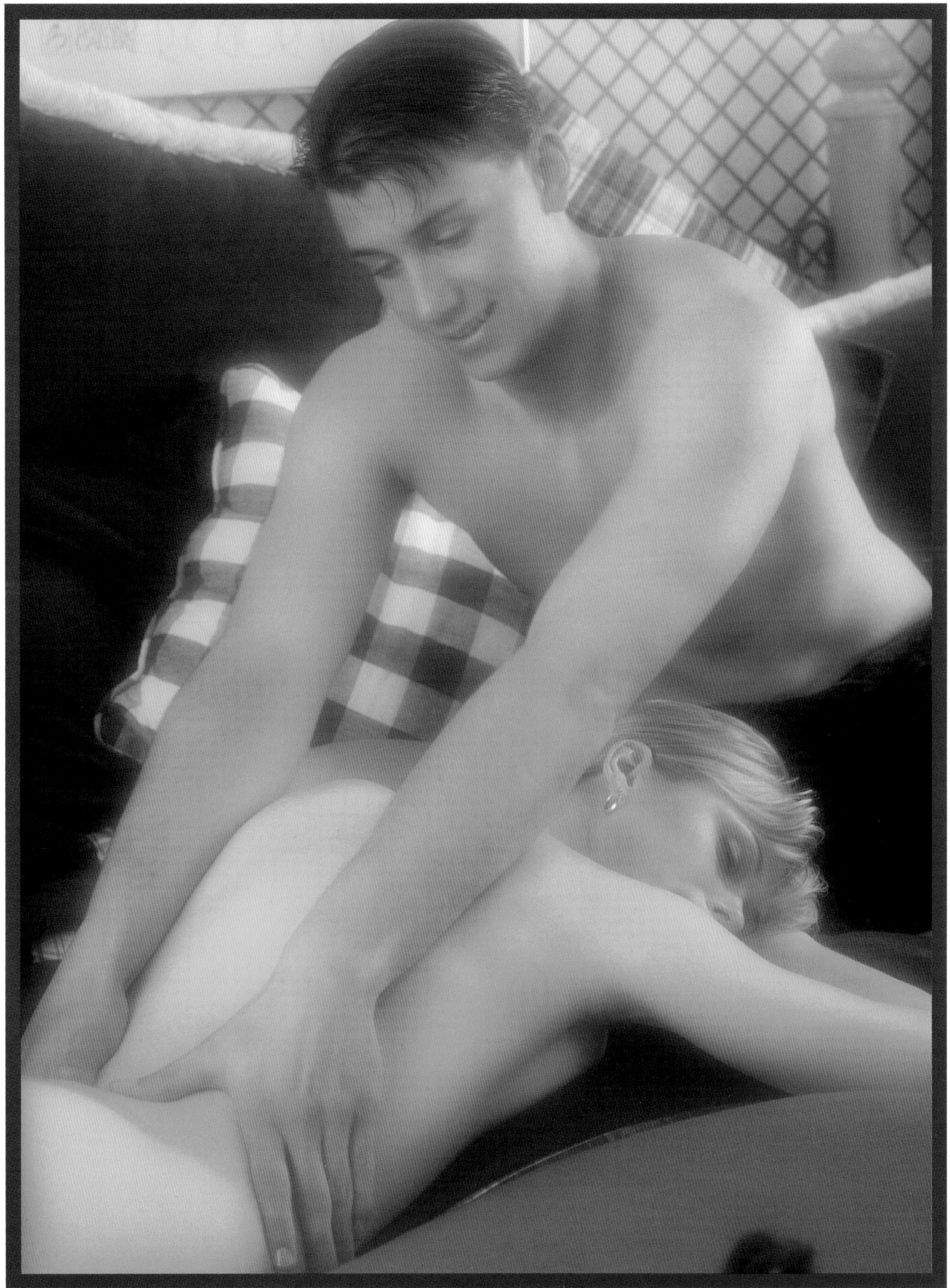

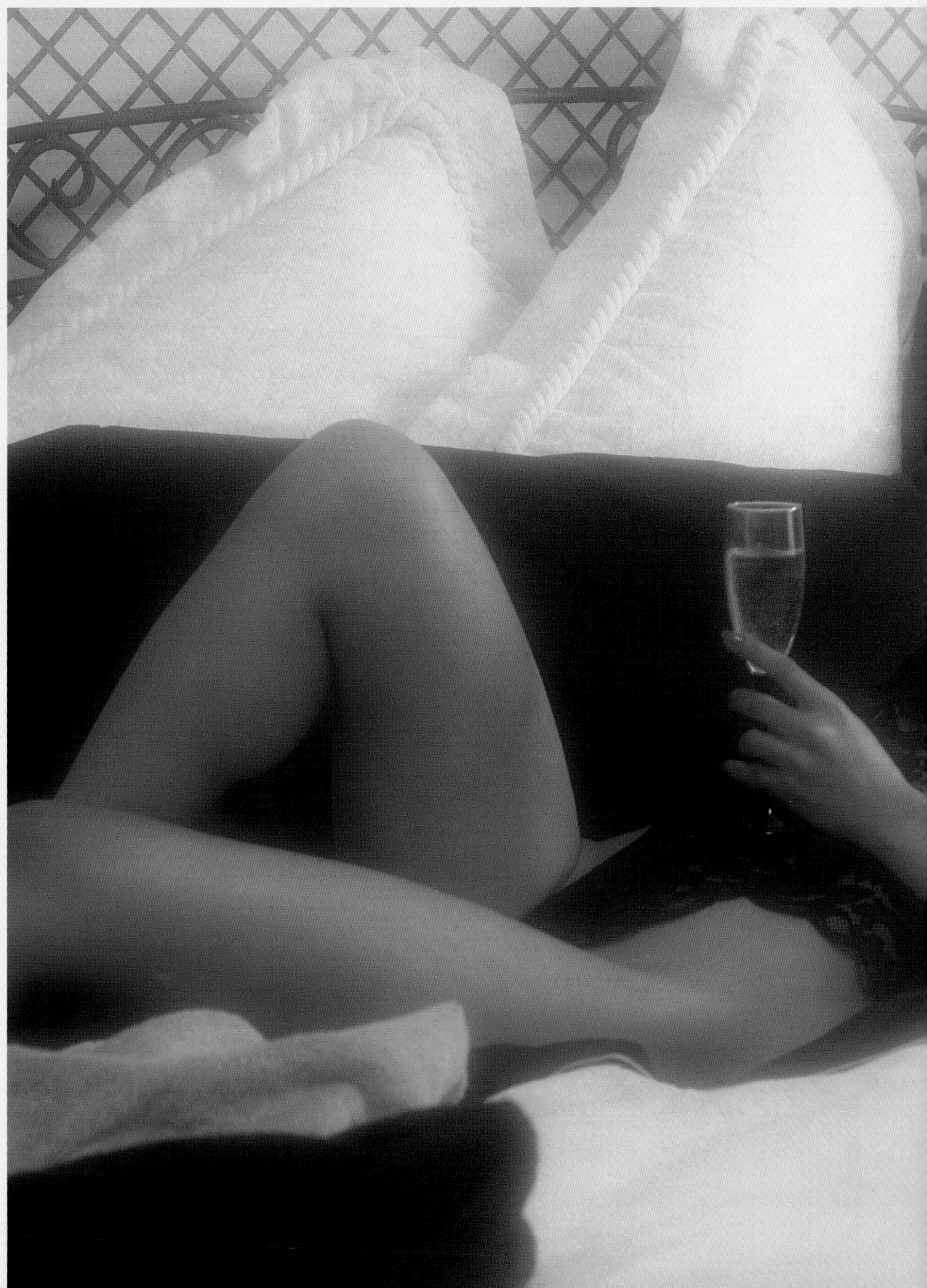

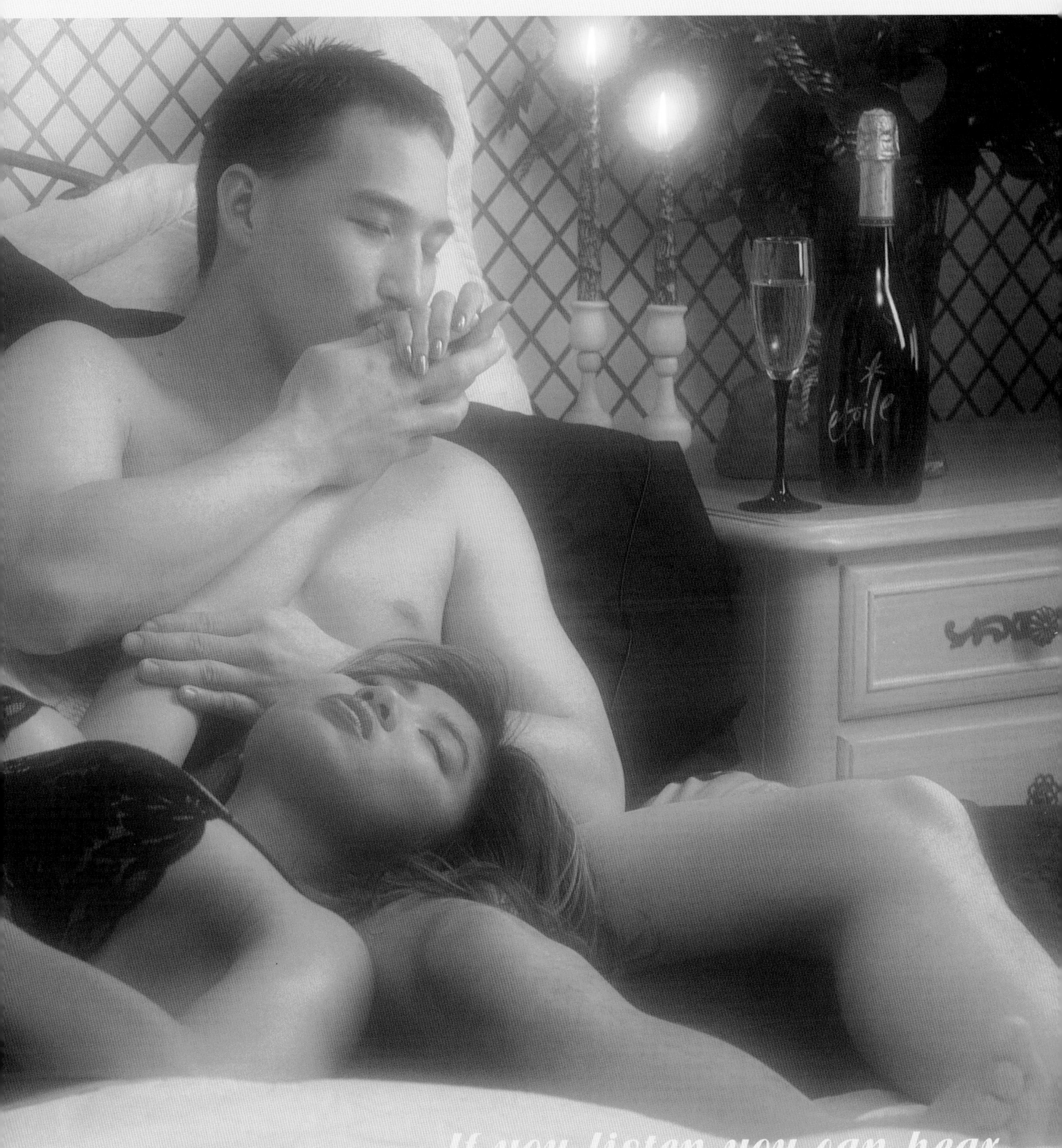

If you listen you can hear your lover's sighs of contentment, you can sense their thoughts, you can make the contact even more intimate.

chapter three

Ambiance

A perfect setting for romantic massage will help ensure the time you want to enjoy with your lover will be tranquil, peaceful, and sensual. It is called "Ambiance" — that special atmosphere or mood created by a particular environment.

When giving a romantic massage, it is important that everything be just right. Giving and receiving massage is wonderfully relaxing, and using just a few simple guidelines to prepare for that special moment will result in a beautiful experience together. Follow these steps to ensure a sensually fantastic time.

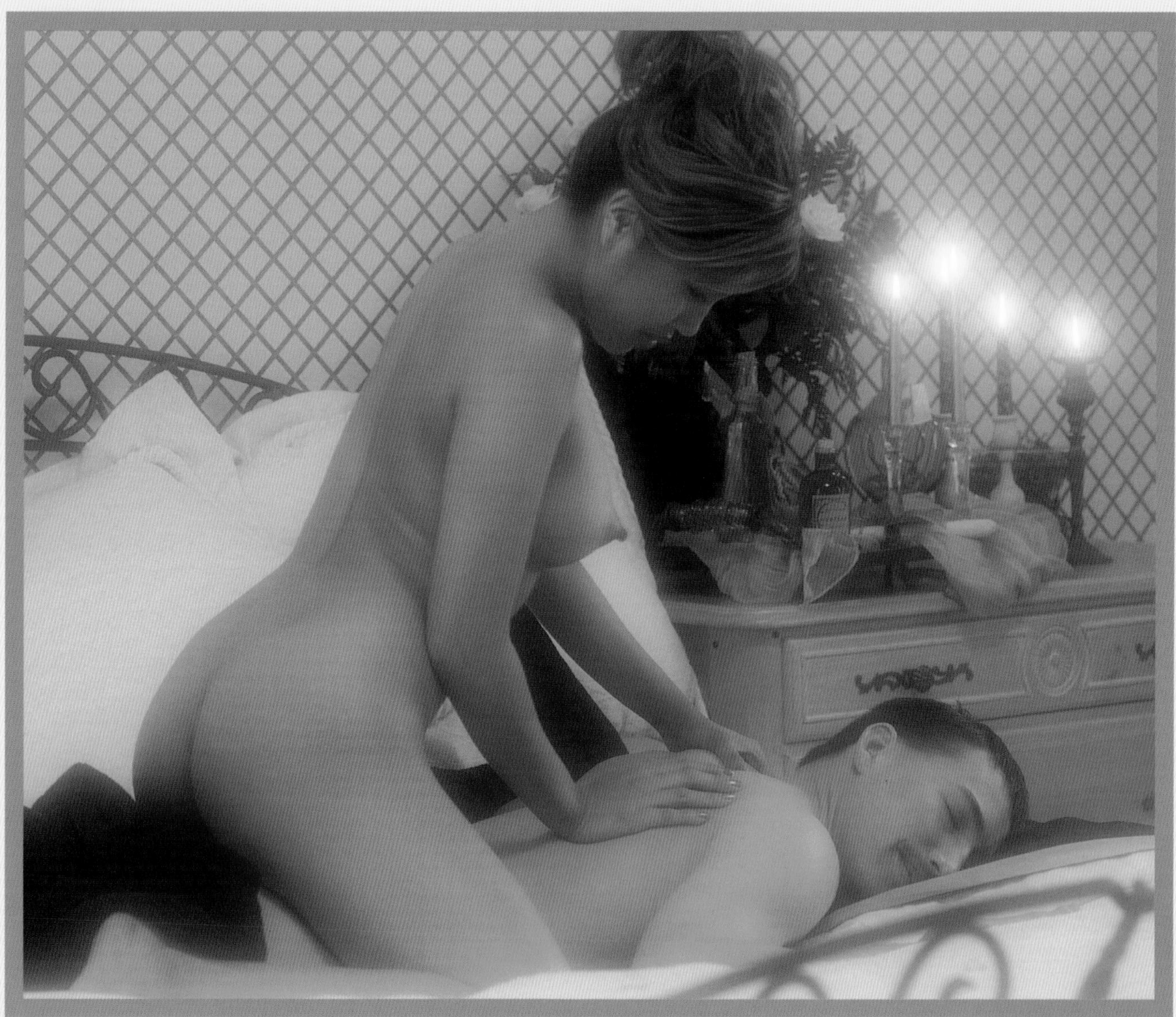

Room Temperature

Keep the room you have chosen for massage at a comfortably warm temperature (75 ° F./24 ° C.). Eliminate any drafts. Usually romantic massage is given with both lovers unrobed, unless of course wearing sensuous underclothing or lingerie is part of your playful time together.

As your partner's body is massaged, its temperature lowers as they become still and relaxed. Making your partner warm, comfortable, and relaxed is essential to an enjoyable time.

Indirect Lighting

Choosing the appropriate room lighting is also very important in setting the right mood. Bright or harsh lighting should be avoided, it often inhibits feelings of intimacy.

If an intimate time is planned during daylight hours, draw the curtains or lower the shades to create subdued shadows. Otherwise, indirect, dimmed incandescent lights work very well. Candles or oil lamps are excellent and provide a much softer effect in the room.

Illumination should be just enough to make out images, but too dark to read comfortably. In fact, some people enjoy doing a massage in the dark; this inhibits the sense of sight, but enhances the pleasure of touch.

Quiet Sanctuary

If surrounding noises are a common occurrence, plan for quiet. Local hotels, bed and breakfasts, or resorts occasionally have weekend, midweek, or off-season special rates on rooms. Escape to a place that is quiet, guarantees no interruptions, pampers you both, and promises very special memories. It may convey the feeling of splurging or having a tryst.

If leaving home is not an option, try to keep loud noises to a minimum. If neighbors have loud parties every Friday night or mow lawns on Saturday mornings, choose Thursday evenings or Saturday afternoons as your private time.

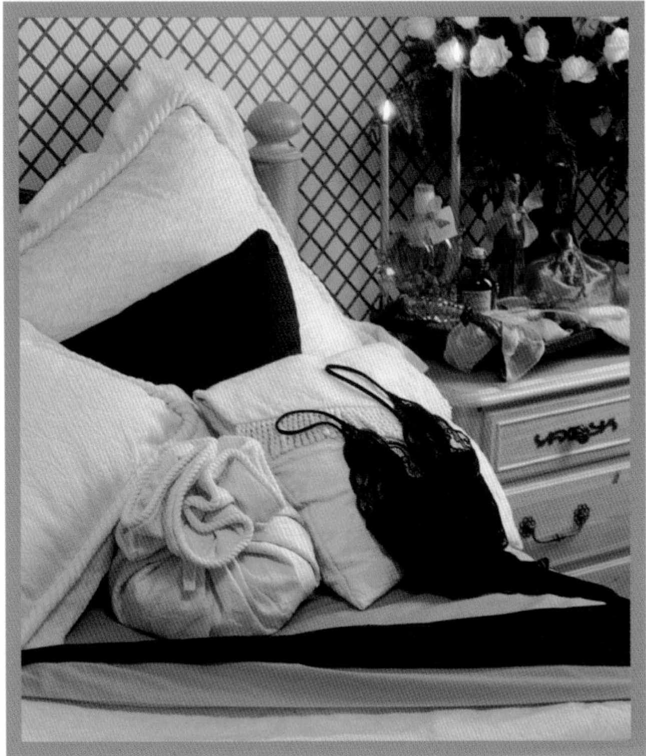

Soft, indirect lighting sets the mood for romance.

Play your partner's favorite soft music. A long cassette tape or CD on continuous play will ensure no distractions. Music can definitely enhance the seductive mood while muffling any unavoidable sounds.

Sometimes just peace and quiet are preferred. That's quite all right. The sound of skin massaging skin, long cleansing breaths or sighs, the rhythm of heart beats, the soft low moans of pleasure and relaxation that accompany each massage stroke can be beautiful music indeed. Even a breeze rustling through the trees, distant wind chimes, or quiet water fountains can add to this symphony of sounds.

Always be prepared for the moment:

- ♥ *Aromatic candles*
- ♥ *Bottle of champagne*
- ♥ *Romantic greeting card*
- ♥ *Romantic music*
- ♥ *Special gift of lingerie*

No Interruptions

I once saw a unique "do not disturb" sign for the honeymoon suite at a hotel. It said, "***Please, do not interruptus!***" And, humorous as it was, it did get the point across quite well. The point being, it is difficult to get into, much less maintain, a romantic mood when there are interruptions.

Distractions that destroy any chance at romance include: telephones, answering machines, pagers, pets, children, knocks at the door, or loud noises. Plan ahead for these little inconveniences. Check the pets, tuck the kids in, and lock the doors. The sensuality of the moment, whether massage is a prelude to romantic things or innocent sensual exploration and teasing, can disappear instantly with any unexpected interruptions. Part of a beautiful time alone with your lover is getting away from the distractions of the world and your normal daily routine.

Proper Body Support

When giving a massage, the proper surface depends on the effect you are trying to create. Deeper, stronger strokes require a firm surface; possibly the floor with a duvet, comforter, or thick blankets. *(Make certain to provide enough padded surface to kneel on.)* For medium pressure strokes, a futon or extra firm

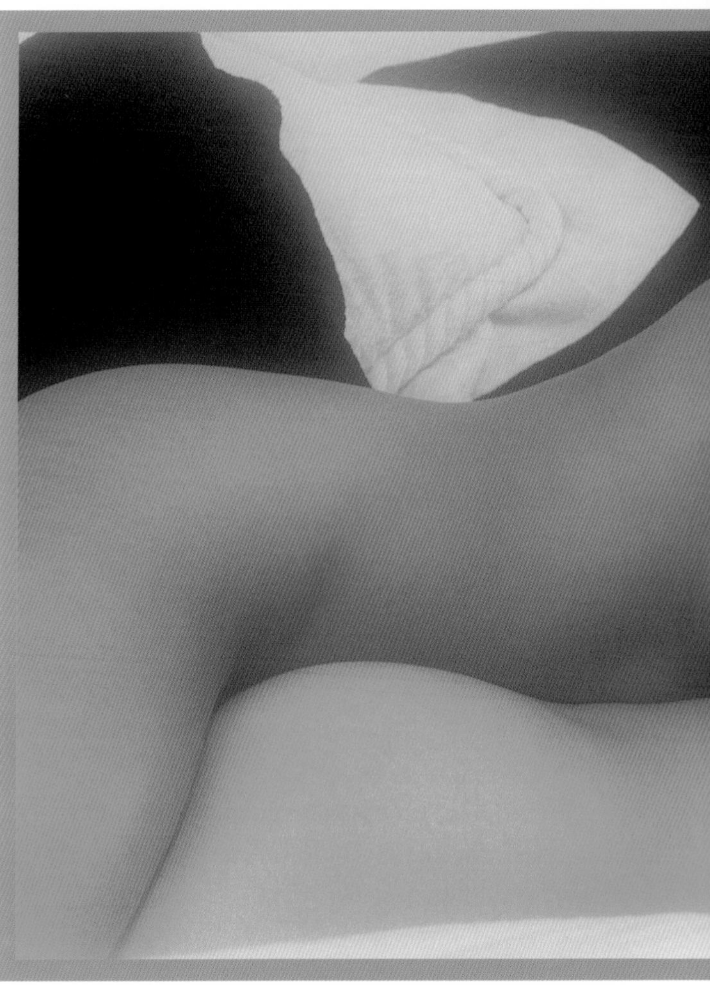

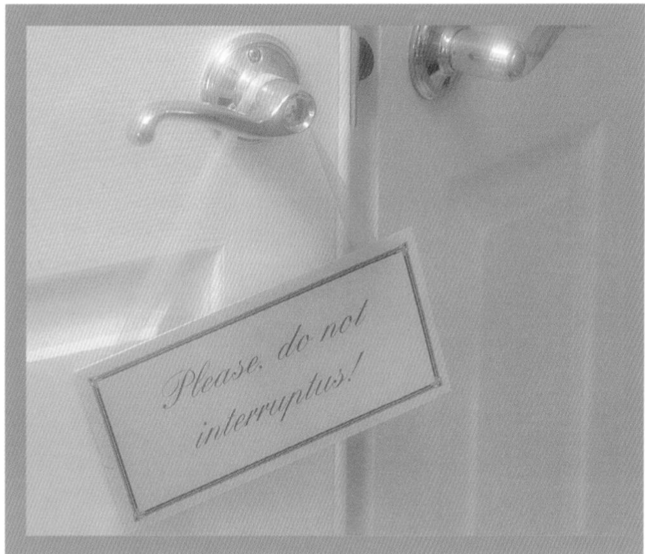

Hang a sign that informs others of your private time.

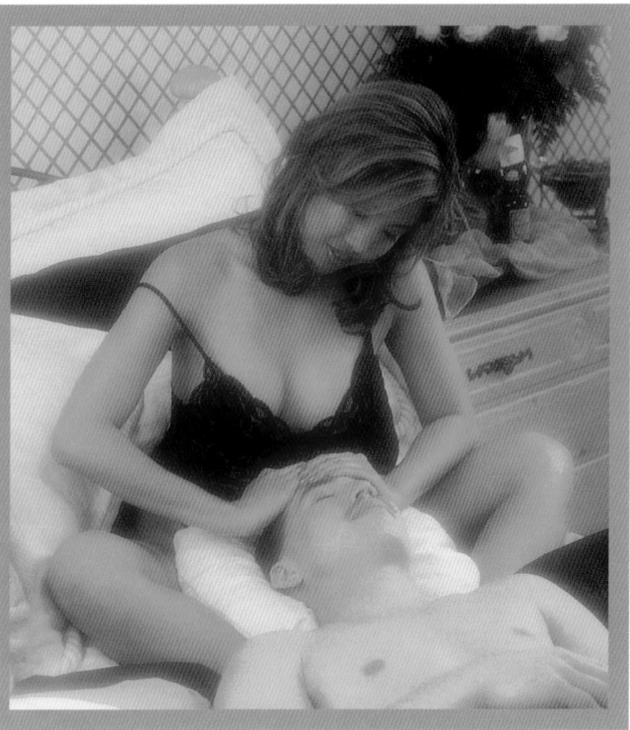

Extra pillows and towels can keep your lover comfortable.

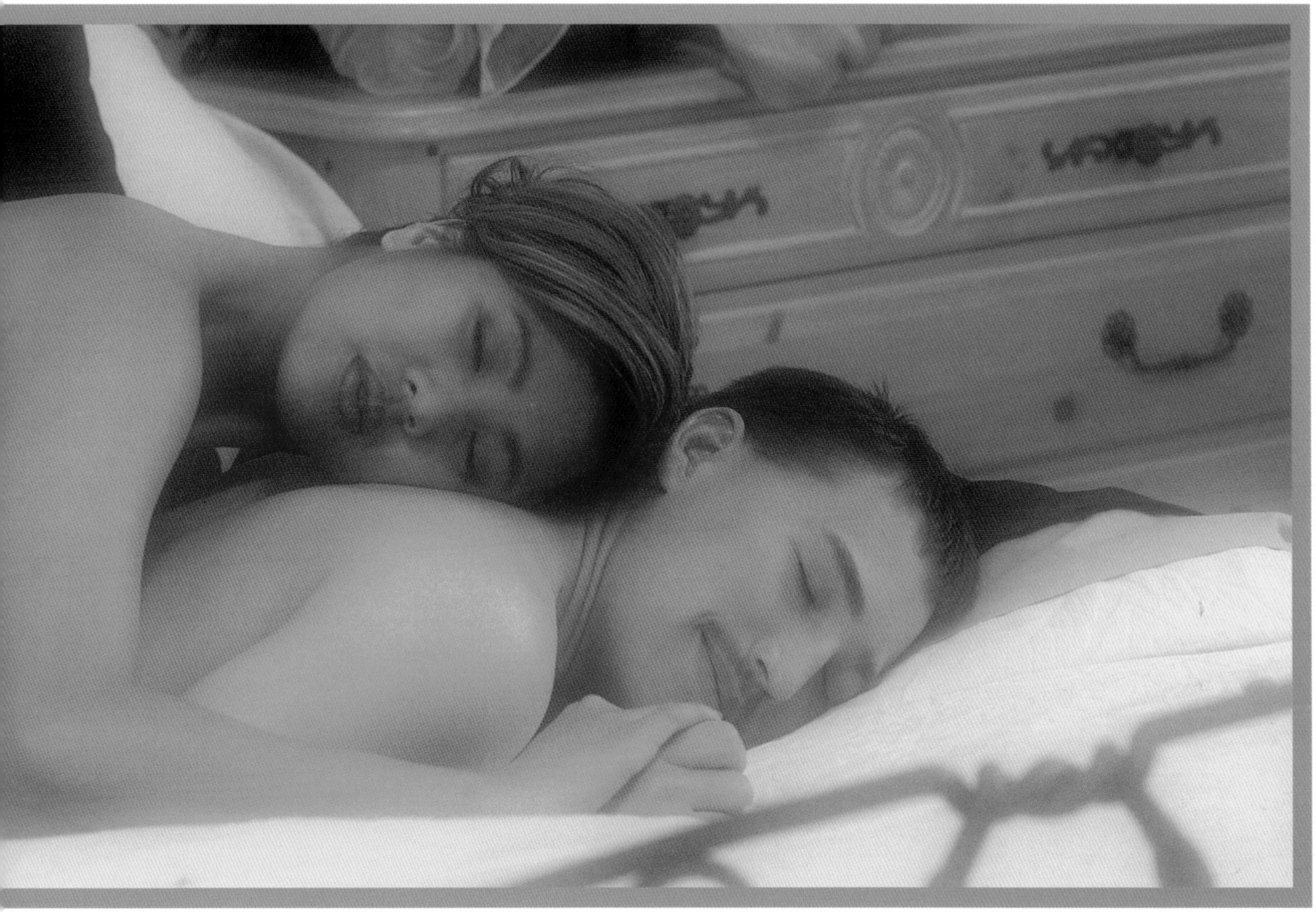

support mattress should suffice. For the lighter strokes of romance, any bed mattress ought to be just fine.

Have extra pillows to support the neck or legs and towels or blankets to wrap around your partner in case of chill. It is impossible for muscles to relax if they are uncomfortable.

Hands & Hygiene

Smell can also have a definite effect on the outcome of a romantic massage. Be certain to not only bathe or shower beforehand, but do so with soaps, oils, and splashes that relax and enhance the body. Hands should be clean and soft. Accidental scratches or scrapes can be avoided when nails are clipped and filed to a smooth edge, and jewelry is removed.

Clothing and jewelry can be important enhancements, distractions, or frustrations during massage. Part of setting a romantic mood is choosing the right bedroom attire. Flannels or tightly buttoned full length outfits can take away from the spontaneity of the moment. It takes too long to remove complicated clothing or to find the clasp on unwanted jewelry.

Brief silk or lace lingerie sets the mood for a romantic interlude. And, if the room is an inviting temperature, no clothing whatsoever is enjoyable, too. The important thing to be certain of, is that you and your partner feel comfortable at all times. If either of you is shy, start with some clothing or covering. As you relax, clothes or covers can be removed.

Guide your lover to your location by using candles to light a path from the front door to where you are waiting.

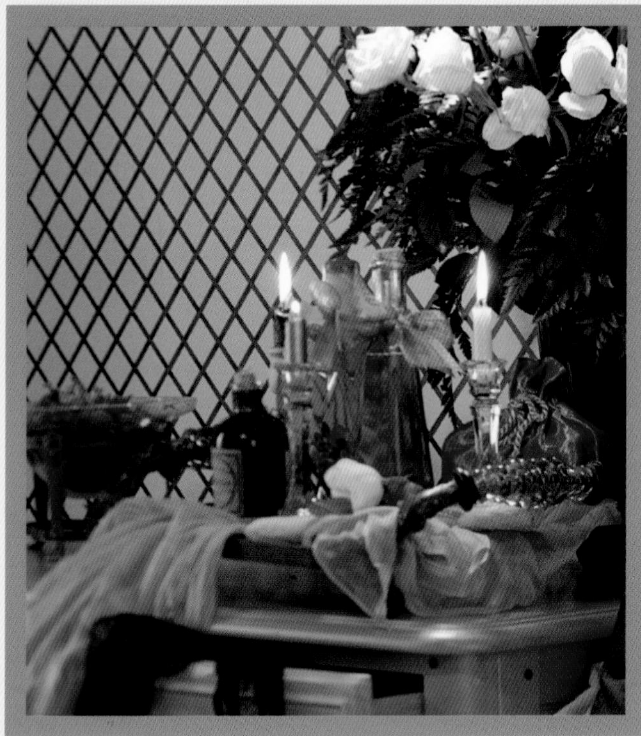

Oils & Essences

Oils are usually the best choice for both skin lubrication and moisturizing. Lotions are water based with waxes and are good for moisturizing dry skin, but lose their lubricating qualities quickly (30 to 60 seconds). Creams are petroleum, wax, and lanolin based. They feel thick and greasy, and usually do not absorb well (10 minutes or more).

Natural carrier oils, on the other hand, lubricate efficiently, are light to the touch, and absorb readily (several minutes). Some excellent carrier oils are: almond (sweet), apricot kernel, avocado, extra light olive, sunflower, or a light vegetable oil. Oils can stain clothing and sheets and go rancid over time; so take precautions and launder appropriately. A carrier oil is important, it dilutes essential oils and protects the skin from irritation. Choose a carrier oil with very little or no scent. Its blending with essential oils for their specific qualities of scent can enhance the massage, in unexpected ways.

Essential oils can be found at boutiques, health food stores, spas, or bath supply stores. Call first to check prices and see if the supplier has premixed blends. Essential oils are highly concentrated aromatic oils that have been extracted from flowers, herbs, leaves, seeds, and/or plant roots. They not only have medical qualities, but the romantic qualities of relaxation (sedative), relief of muscle tension (antispasmodic, anesthetic, analgesic), the increase of blood flow (circulatory stimulant), and sexual enhancement (aphrodisiac). If you choose to blend oils rather than purchase them premixed, certain combinations are listed below:

Aphrodisiac Blend #1

- ♥ 3 drops ylang-ylang
- ♥ 4 drops sandalwood
- ♥ 4 drops jasmine or rose
- ♥ 1 oz. carrier oil

Aphrodisiac Blend #2

- ♥ 6 drops cedarwood
- ♥ 4 drops lavender
- ♥ 4 drops grapefruit
- ♥ 1 oz. carrier oil

Aphrodisiac Blend #3

- ♥ 6 drops jasmine
- ♥ 4 drops neroli
- ♥ 1 oz. carrier oil

Relaxing Blend #1

- ♥ 6 drops chamomile
- ♥ 4 drops lavender
- ♥ 3 drops orange, bergamot, or grapefruit
- ♥ 1 oz. carrier oil

Relaxing Blend #2

- ♥ 6 drops marjoram
- ♥ 4 drops lavender
- ♥ 4 drops rose or geranium
- ♥ 1 oz. carrier oil

Setting Your Mood

Now that everything is prepared for an intimate time of romantic massage, you and your partner should be ready too. Massage feels great, even the first time. Although your technique is not perfect, the massage is going to be enjoyed and appreciated. People love being touched. Make your strokes unhurried and fluid to relax and satisfy your lover. If you listen closely, you can hear your partner's moans of contentment and bliss. You can almost sense their thoughts, the contact is so close and intimate.

The one receiving a massage, needs to do only one thing: let go of tension and enjoy every moment, every stroke, every sensation. Trust your partner to pamper every need and satisfy every desire. The one giving a massage should anticipate the partner's wants and desires, attend to them, and make it a pleasurably romantic, if not erotic, experience. Follow the contours of their body; remain in constant contact with them. Imagine your hands gliding effortlessly over every nook and cranny, each swell and rise, every hollow and eddy. Sense what they feel. Tease and explore. This is not meant to be a massage from a professional practitioner. This is an intimate, personal massage between lovers, intended to give pleasure and sensual satisfaction.

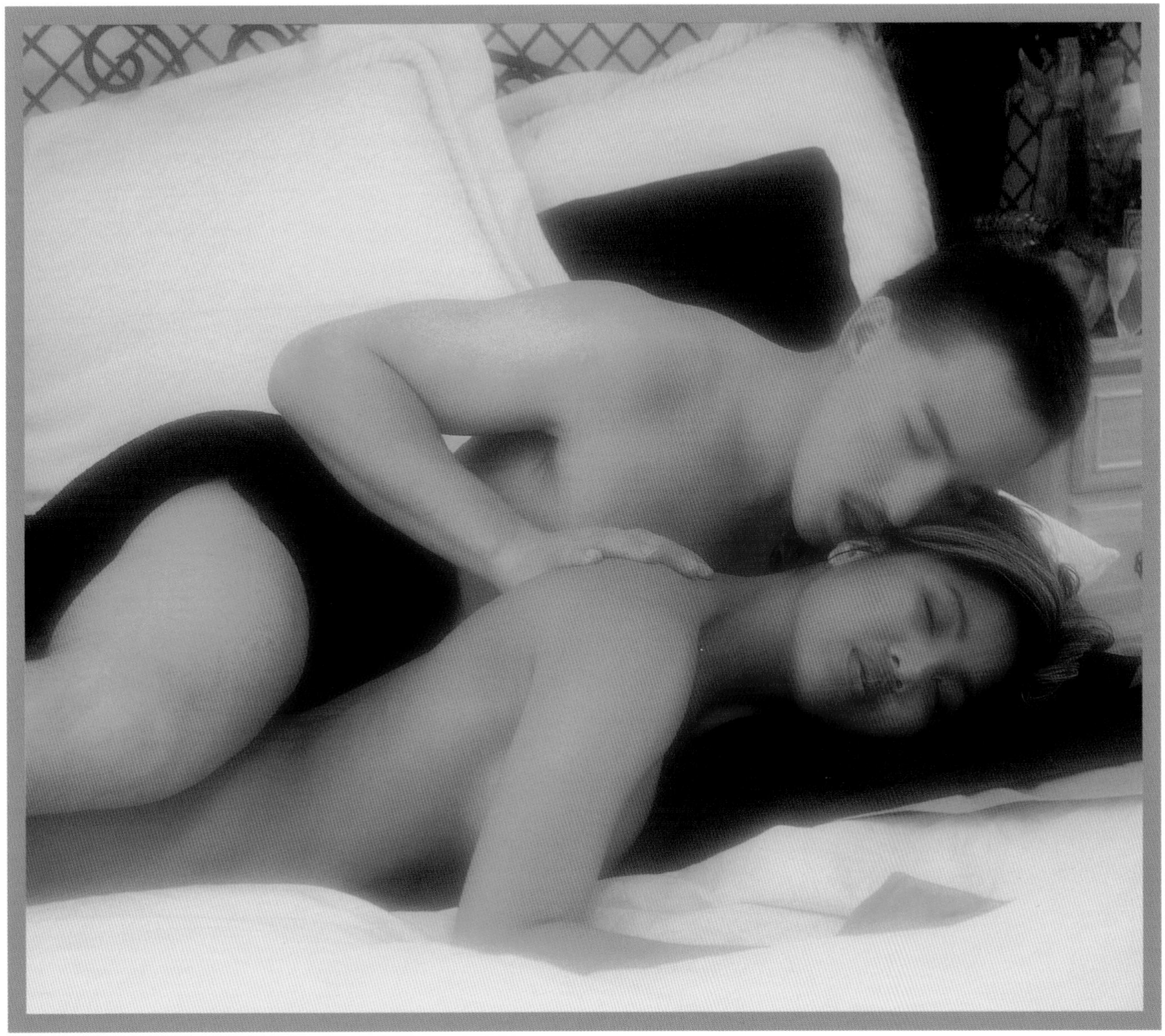

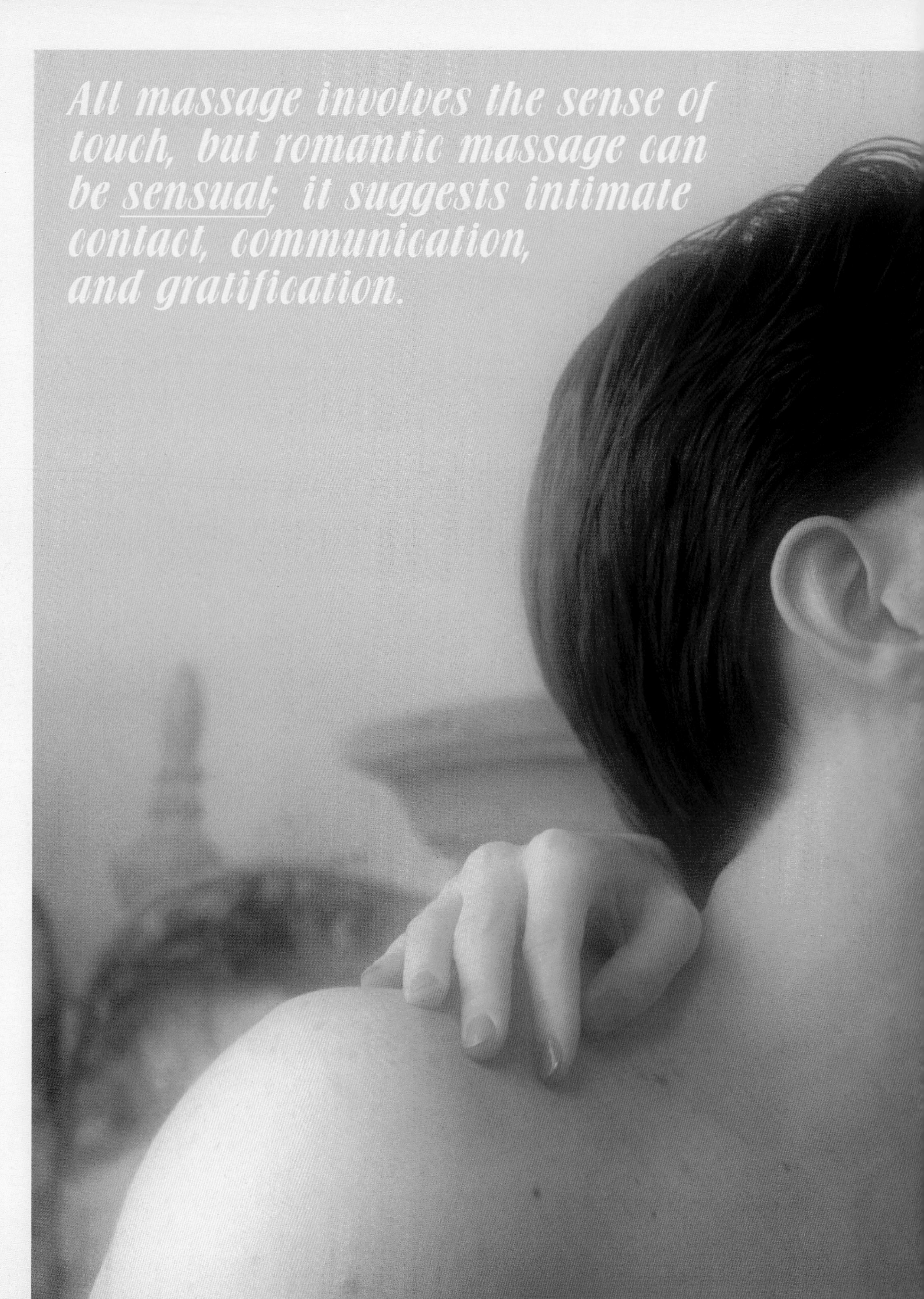

All massage involves the sense of touch, but romantic massage can be sensual; it suggests intimate contact, communication, and gratification.

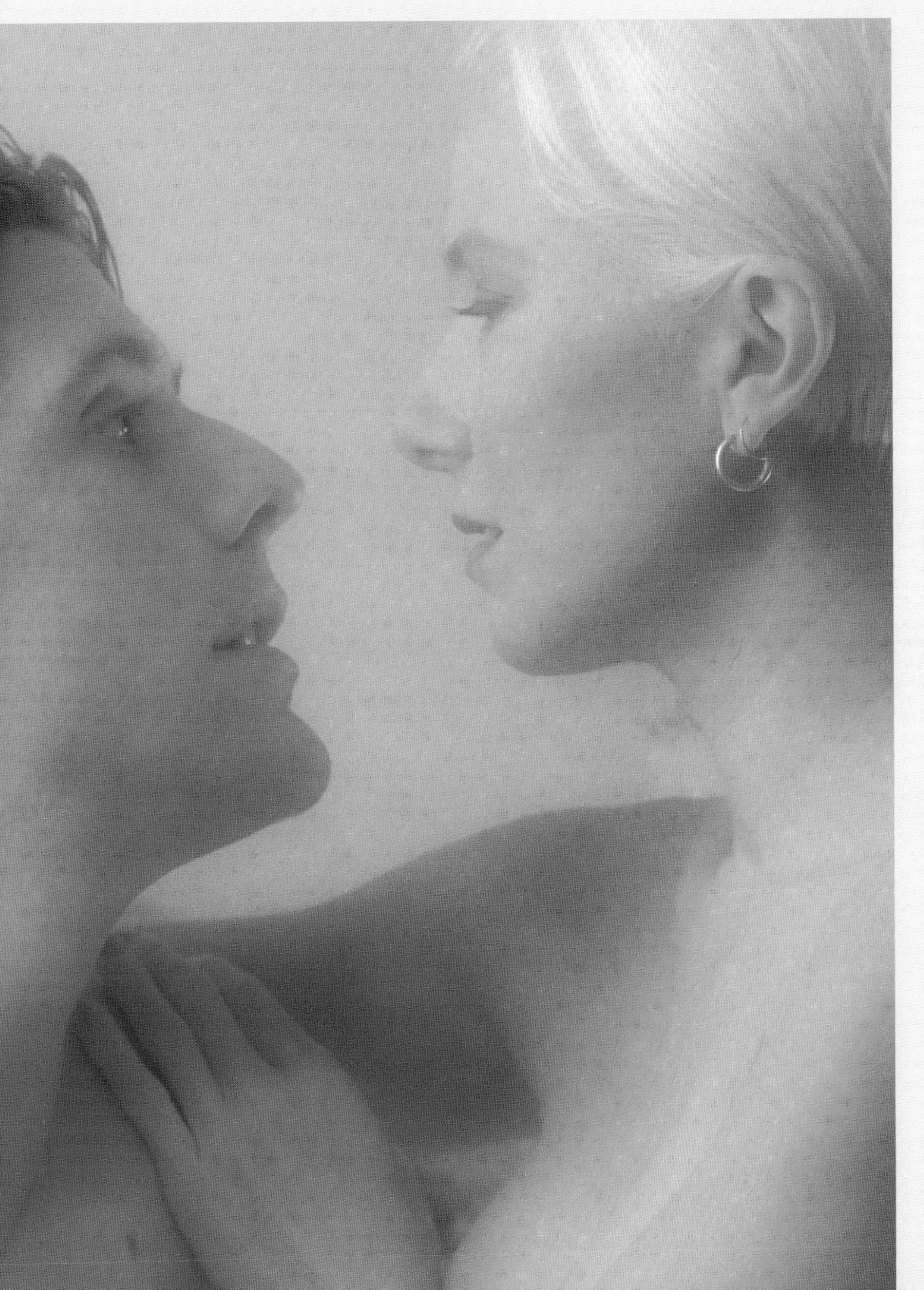

chapter four

Different Strokes

All massage involves the sensation of touch, but certain types of massage are more sensuous in nature suggesting intimate contact, communication, and gratification. *Romantic* massage deals both with relaxation and arousal of sexual feelings. This may sound contradictory at first, but frequently a person must be relaxed to feel comfortable before being open to the possibility of being intimate with someone.

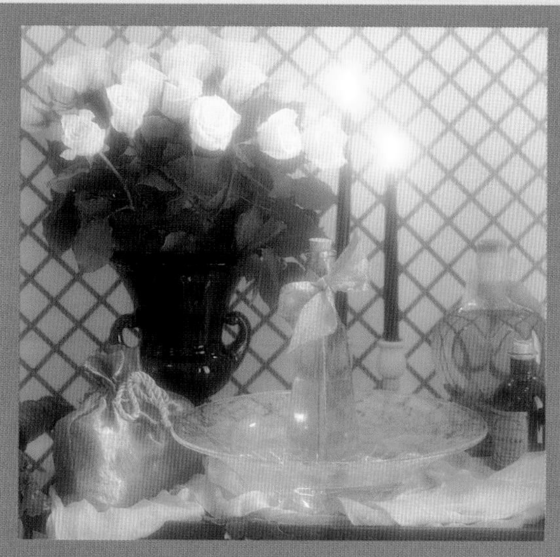

Warming massage oil in a bowl of hot water approximately 120 ° F./49 ° C. helps warm the hands as well as your partner's body.

Application of Oil

Prior to beginning sensual and romantic massage, the skin must be oiled; this will enhance several areas as well as lubricate to minimize friction. Some friction is good because it creates heat to warm muscles, but too much friction on the skin can be uncomfortable; this is why oils are preferred over lotions or creams. Oils lubricate well and absorb within minutes, which allows some friction to occur while warming the skin. Using the following sequence will ensure a successful massage:

- ♥ Apply ½–1 teaspoon of oil to palm of the hand.
- ♥ Rub hands together to lubricate and warm.
- ♥ Massage your partner's body using light, long strokes to apply oil and lubricate skin.
- ♥ Repeat the above steps as needed.

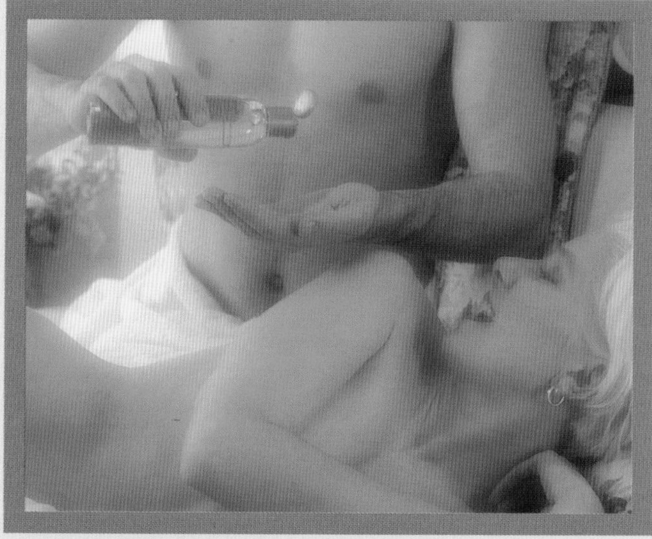

Lubricate both hands with ½–1 teaspoon of oil, and rub them together to warm them prior to massaging your partner's body.

Choose your partner's favorite love songs, record a tape for romantic background music.

Massage Strokes

Five basic Swedish massage strokes are used in both therapeutic and romantic massage. An array of variations to these five basic strokes can each create pleasure and enjoyment.

Romantic gestures have no hidden agenda. Their main purpose is to express love, to show that she is significant and special to you; to express that you think of him often.

EFFLEURAGE

Effleurage is long, flowing or gliding strokes that are generally soothing and gentle. Effleurage strokes usually cause a profound relaxation of muscles, which allows body fluids to flow easier in vessels throughout the body. These strokes also relax the mind, taking it from an alert or normal brain wave state to a deeper, more restful brain wave state similar to that achieved through meditation or sleep.

Effleurage strokes can be the most sensual and erotic movements in massage. Their flowing and continuous motion is both soothing and non-threatening. These strokes are used when applying oil and when moving from one body area to the next. Effleurage is also used to slowly explore and enjoy each area of your lover's body. The effleurage strokes include:

Aura Strokes are long, flowing strokes performed approximately 1–2" above the body. People sensitive to the body's bio-electric energy field (aura) can feel and smooth out variances in the auric field. These may produce impressions such as tingly sensations, differences in heat, or pressure over the body and in the palms of the massage giver's hands.

Feathering is ultralight effleurage strokes using only the fingertips or fingernails. Very light strokes trigger specific neural receptors that can arouse gentle, sensitive moods. If this stroke is executed too quickly, it can feel ticklish.

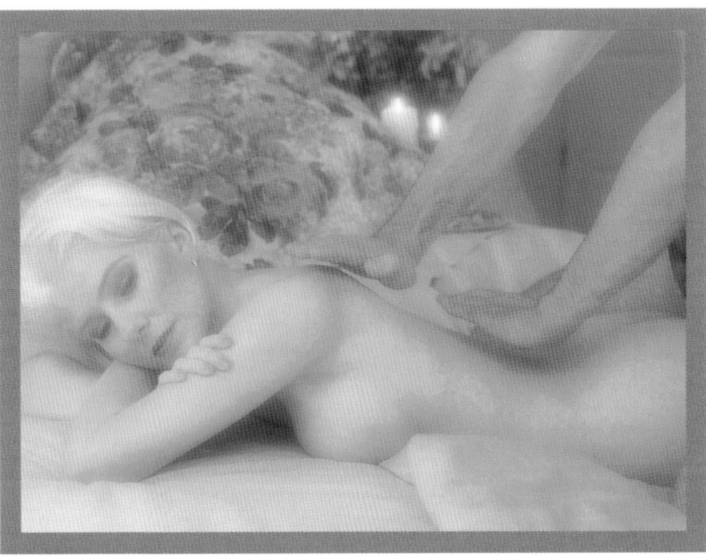

Aura strokes smooth out variances in the body's bio-electric energy field that affect moods and health.

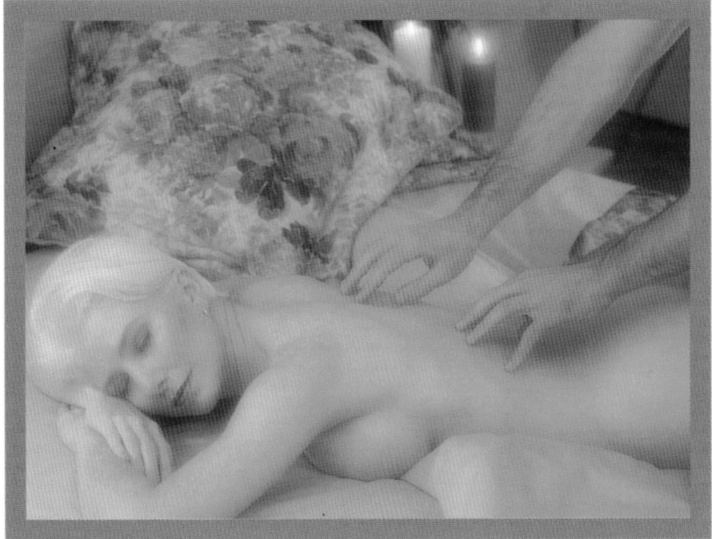

Feathering is an ultralight stroke performed with fingertips and nails that sensitizes nerve endings to evoke sensual feelings in your lover.

Light Effleurage is a long, flowing stroke that uses light pressure. This has a superficial effect; usually gliding over specific areas (windpipe, eyelids, groin) where deeper pressure is not recommended. It is also used when applying oil to minimize friction.

Effleurage encourages the movement of fluids, namely lymph and blood, that carry nutrients to each cell in the body. That is why you should massage toward the heart when working on the arms and legs. This way, you help the natural flow of these vital fluids keep the body functioning correctly.

It is important to keep your hands relaxed and pliable so they conform to the subtle but changing shapes of your partner's body. This stroke offers a wonderfully enjoyable sensation, so, use it liberally over the entire body.

Deep Effleurage is a long, flowing stroke that uses a deeper, more thorough pressure. You may either apply additional pressure with your fingertips while still keeping your hands on the body, or lean your body weight onto your arms. The extra pressure will be distributed over the entire surface of the hand.

This stroke pushes fluids that move toxins and metabolic waste out of tissues. This stroke can be gratifying; especially to people who store stress in certain body areas such as the neck, shoulders, and back.

When muscles become chronically tense from stress, normal blood flow cannot deliver nutrients or remove toxins from tissue cells. Cells fail to function properly, and form knots, aches, and pains. Deep effleurage helps move fluids through these stubborn areas, creating a pleasant sensation.

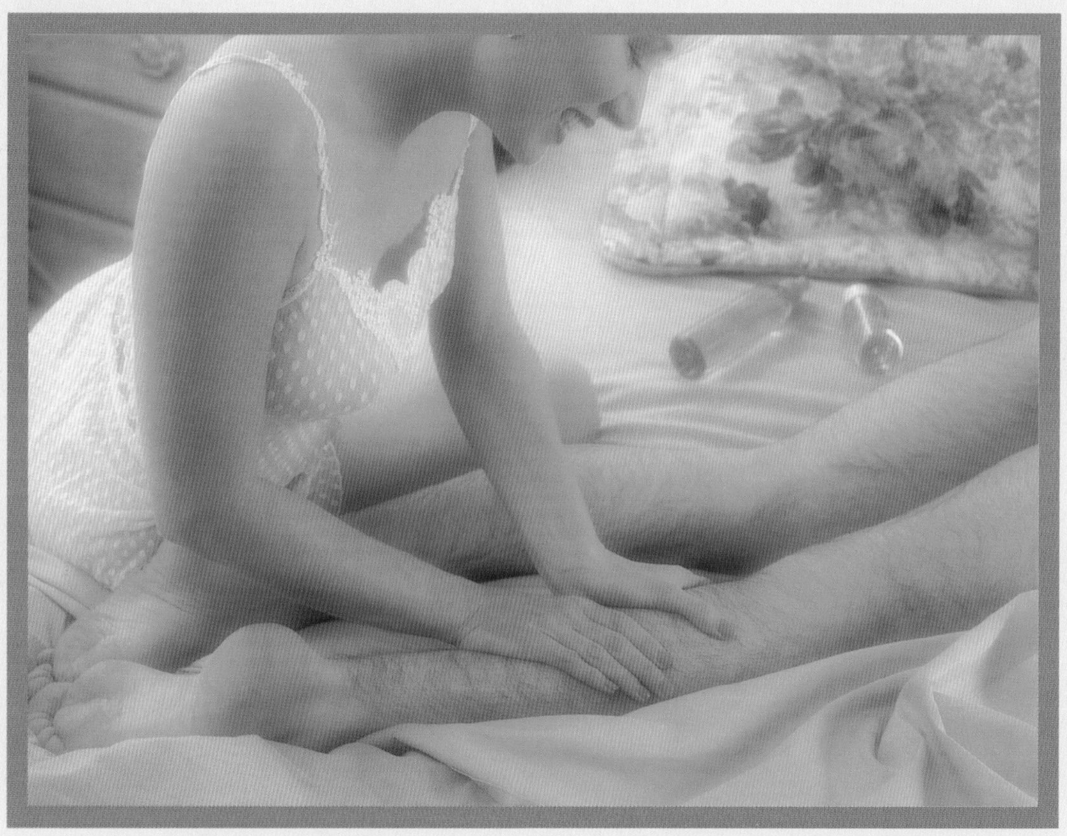

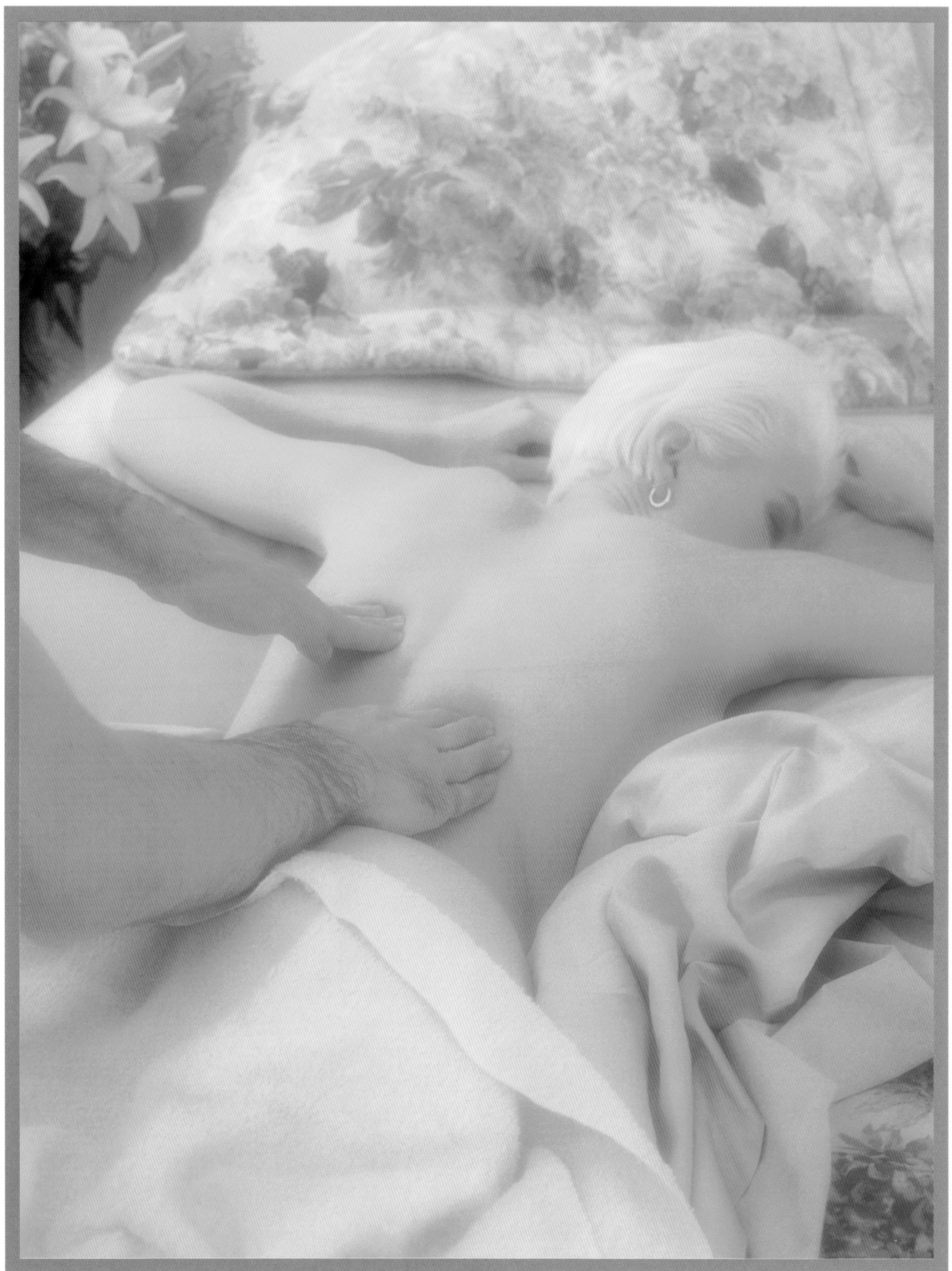

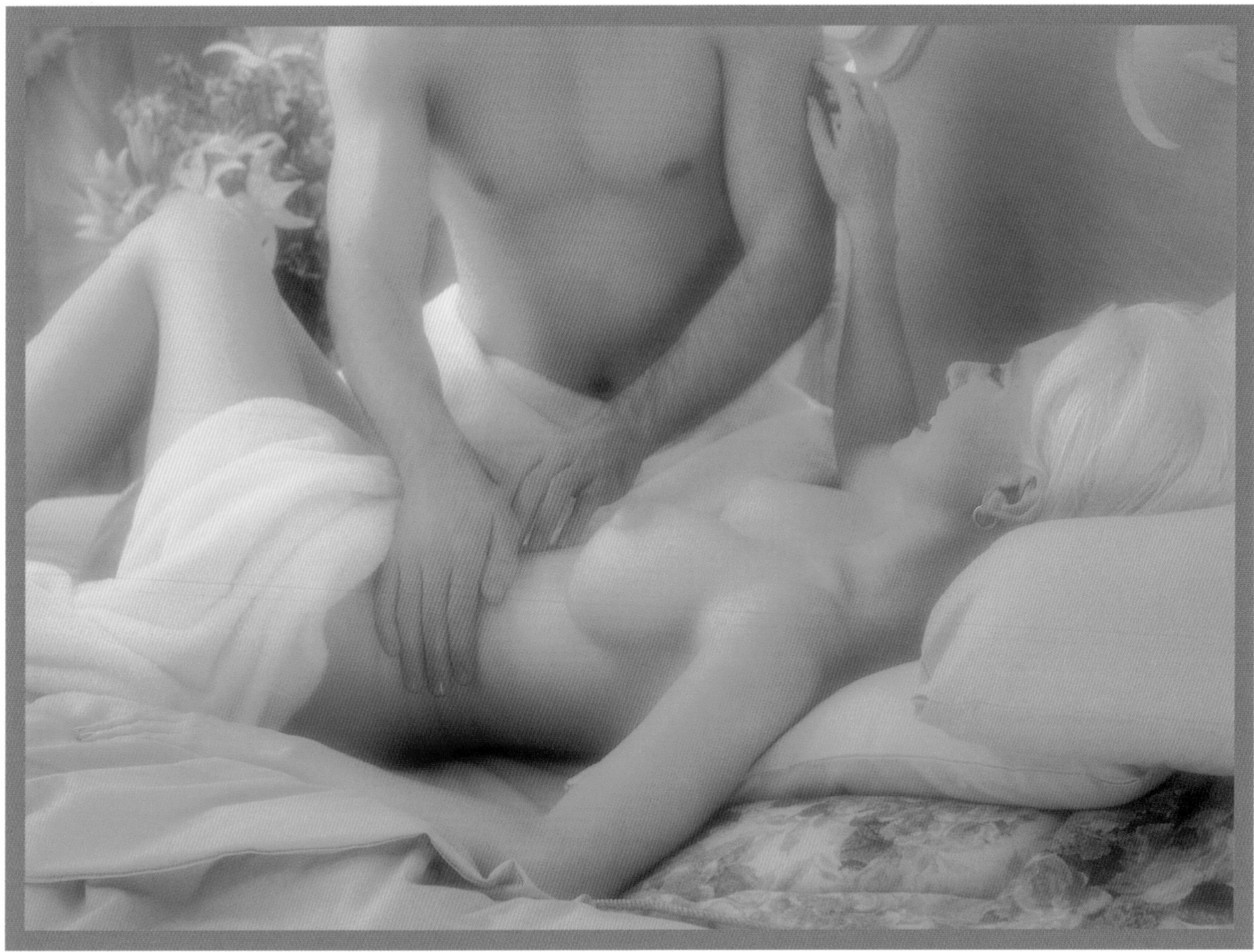

Milking uses long flowing strokes in a continuous motion along the sides of the ribs, waist, and hips.

Milking is a variety of effleurage involving long, flowing strokes along the sides of the body. It is called milking, because the continuous rhythmic pulling movement of the hands on the sides of the ribs, waist, and hips "milks" or squeezes fluids toward other areas of the body.

Milking can be performed while your partner is on their back or stomach. It is an excellent way to relax these often neglected muscles. This stroke accentuates the sensual curves and contours found between the end of the ribs and beginning of the hips.

Kneel to one side of your partner. Place your hand on the body side opposite from your position. Curve your fingers under. As you pull your hand toward you, place your other hand next to where the first hand began. Move in a continuous motion, one hand then the other, slowly traveling up and down this area of the body.

Then, move to the other side of the body and repeat the entire sequence. As your partner lets go of stored tension, you may notice their breathing become slow and deep.

Essential oils whose scents are considered aphrodisiacs are:
♥ Anise ♥ Bois de Rose ♥ Cinnamon ♥ Clary sage ♥ Clove ♥ Ginger ♥ Jasmine ♥ Patchouli ♥ Peppermint ♥ Rose ♥ Sandalwood ♥ Spearmint ♥ Thyme ♥ Ylang ylang

Raking is considered an effleurage stroke because it is long and flowing. It resembles the feathering massage stroke with one difference, raking uses more pressure. Fingers are spread apart like a rake. The stroke is slow and uses medium to firm pressure.

Raking is lusciously teasing before or after deep releasing massage strokes. It is an enjoyable stroke anywhere on the body, but especially after warm soothing strokes.

Rose Milk Silk Bath

2 cups powdered milk
1/2 cup colloidal oatmeal
10 drops rose geranium oil
2 drops peppermint oil
1/2 cup rose water
1 rose in full bloom

Draw the bath. slowly adding powdered milk and colloidal oatmeal. Help dissolve the milk and oatmeal by swirling the water with your hand. Just before you turn off the tap water, add the rose geranium and peppermint oil while swirling the water with your hand.

Before you or your partner steps into the bath, add the rose water. Remove petals from the rose and float them on the surface of the water.

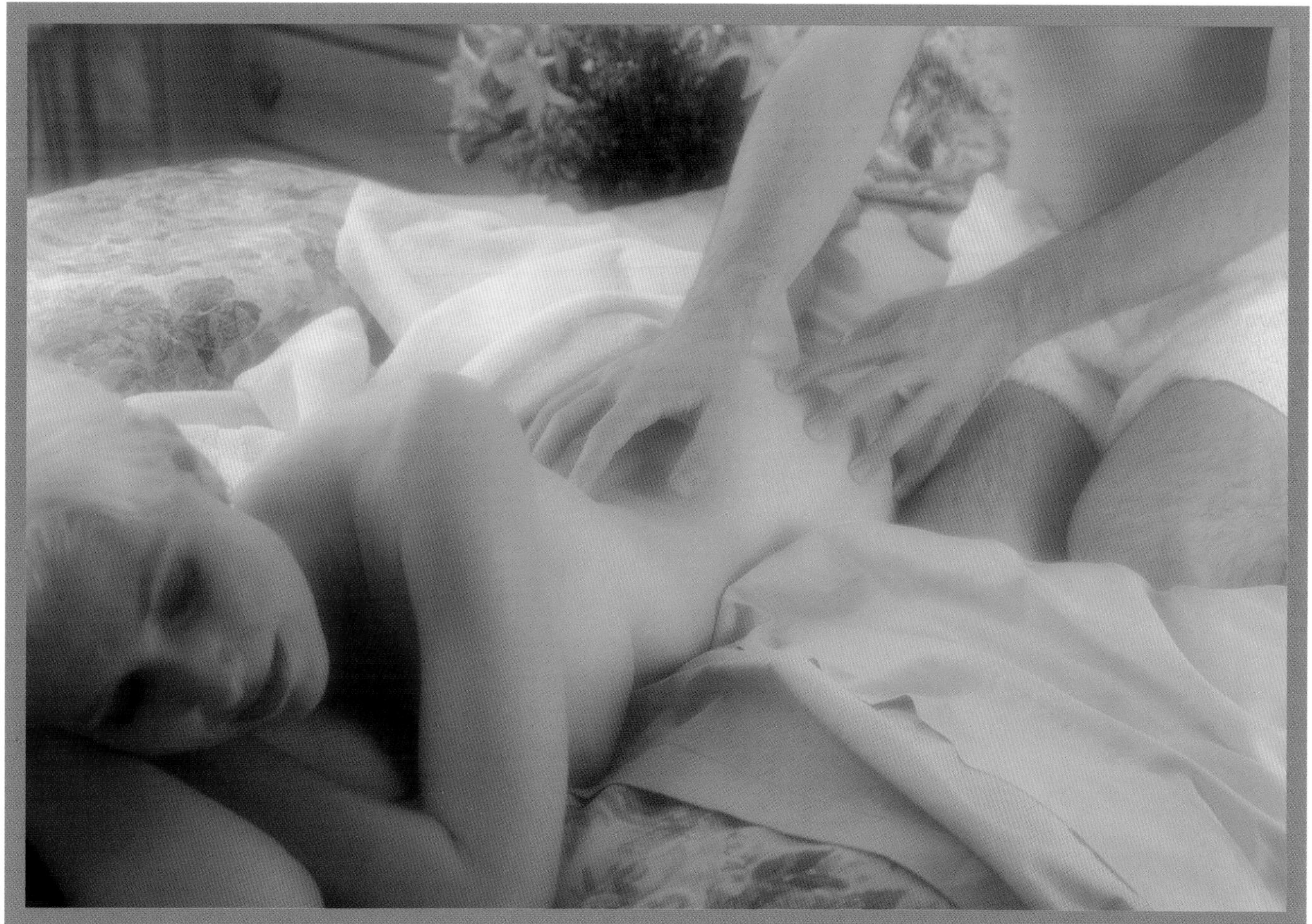

Raking, like feathering, is a stroke performed with fingertips — no nails — that sensitizes nerve endings. This sensitization evokes sensual feelings in your lover. The main difference between feathering and raking is pressure. Raking uses medium to firm pressure, but is slow to avoid tickling response.

Stretching can be a variation of an effleurage stroke. It involves two hands or forearms moving in opposing directions in long, stretching motions. The effect is to lengthen muscles, and when applied to the back, to ease pressure along the length of the spine.

The stroke begins in the center of the area being stretched with either hands or forearms. Medium pressure is applied with some, but not a lot of oil, so there is some friction to the stroke. As the stroke progresses, the hands or forearms continue to the far reaches of the body part; for example, from the center of the back to the neck and buttocks on the far ends.

A **diagonal stretch** is a variation of the basic stretch: one hand is anchored over the bony prominence of the shoulder blade while the other hand moves diagonally toward and over the opposing hip and buttock.

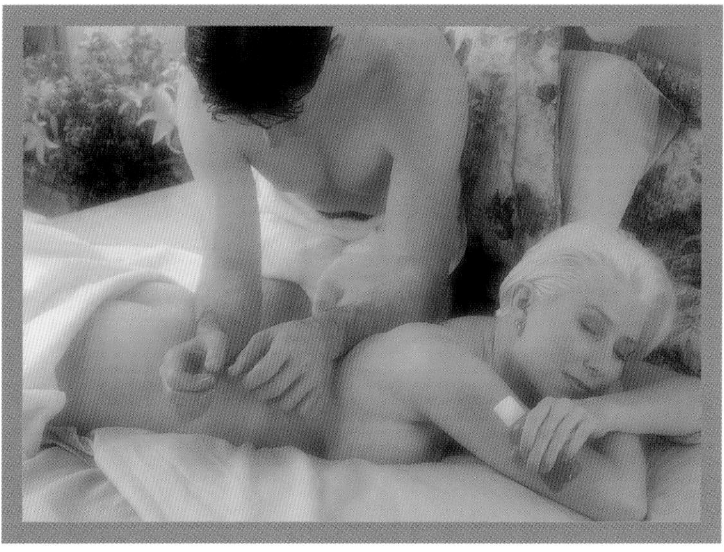

As you begin stretching, your forearms are together with the fleshy portions facing the back and spine. Using bony areas to stroke the spine can be painful.

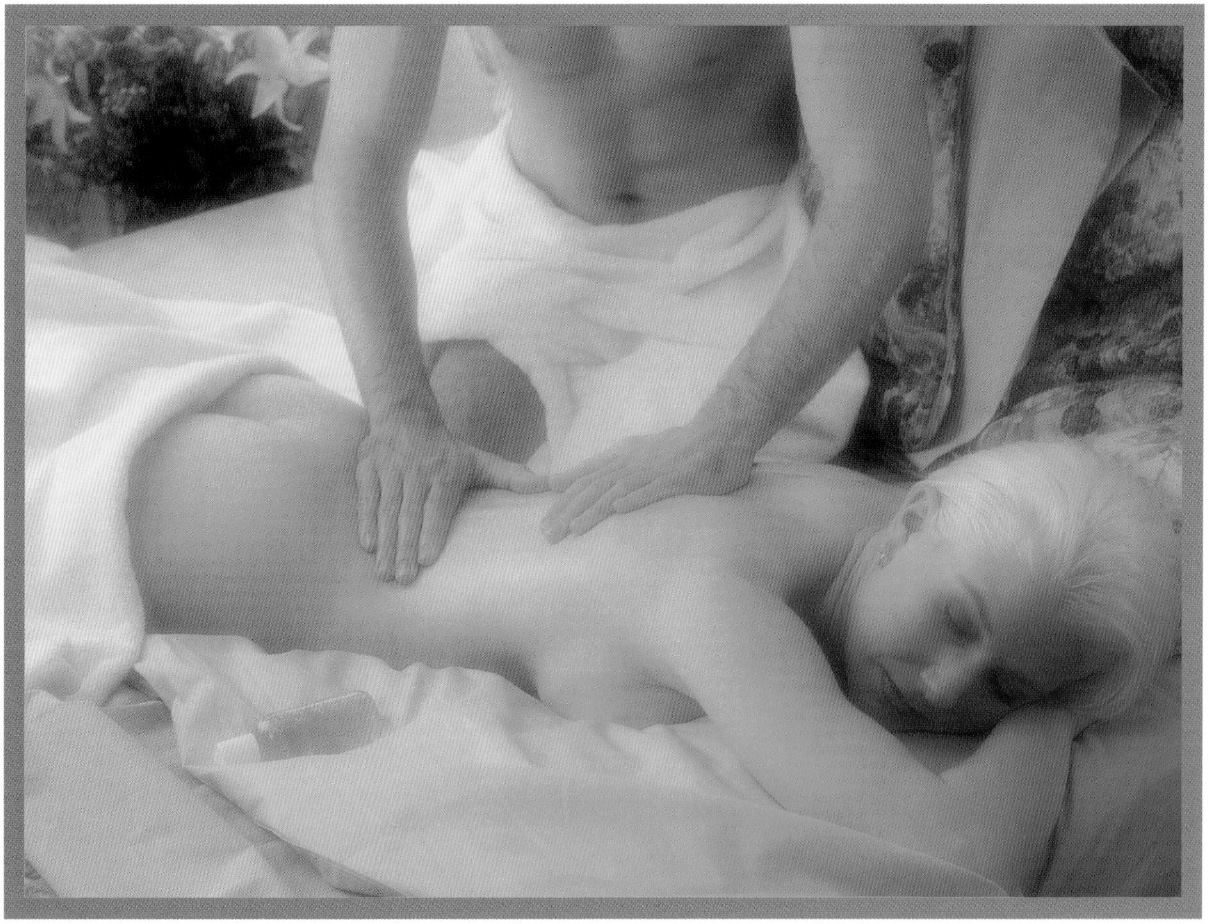

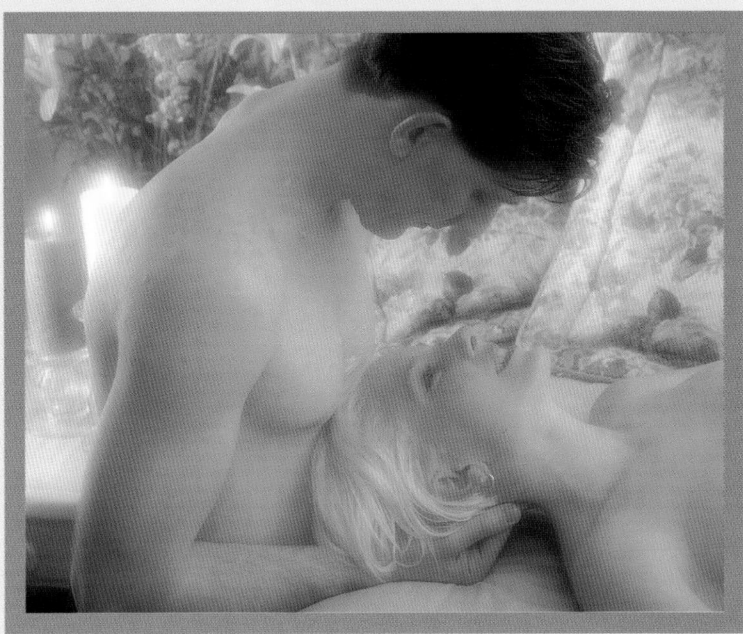

Lifting should be slow and steady. This type of stroke allows your partner to let go as they develop trust in your ability to support them.

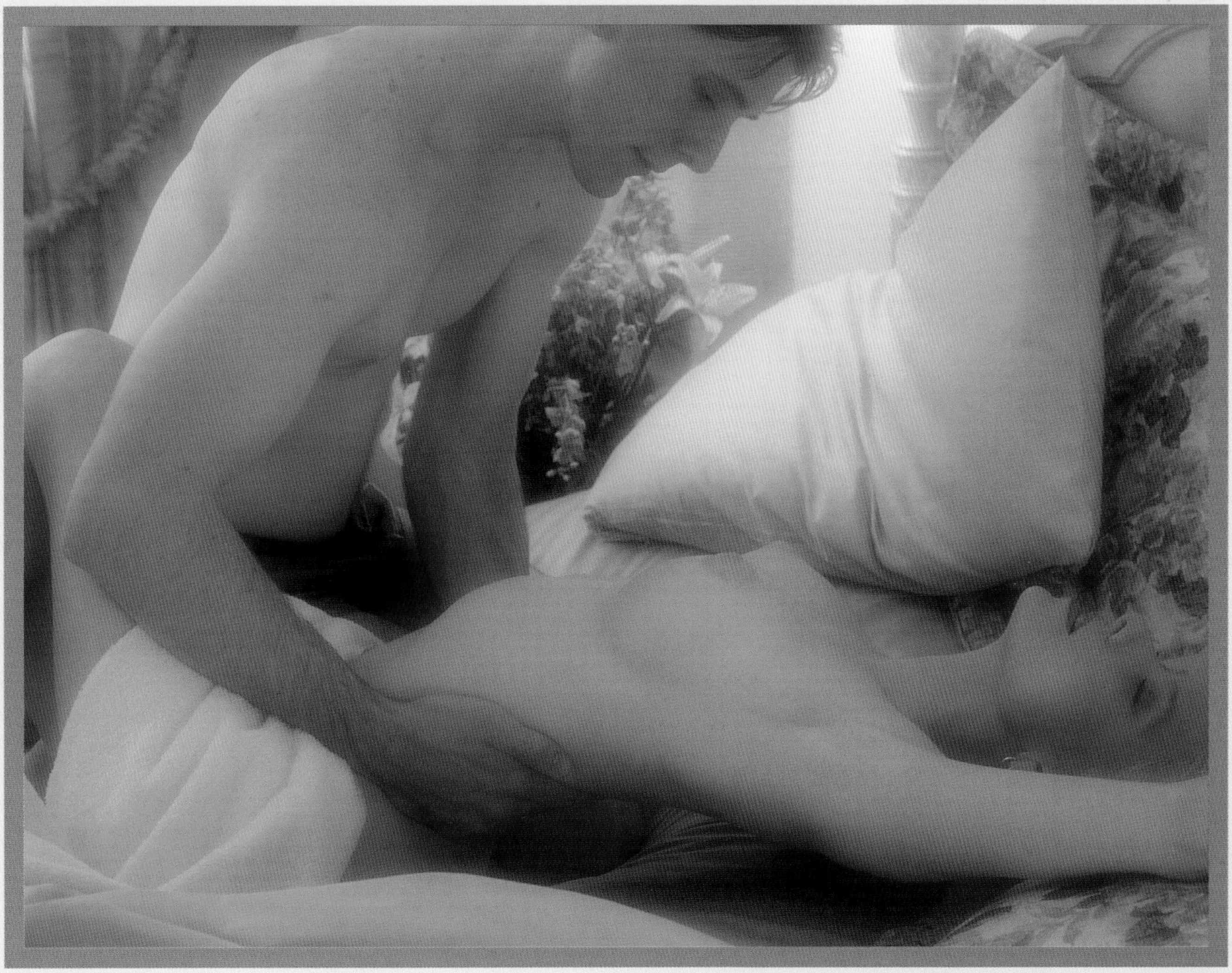

Body Lifts, a last variation of the effleurage stroke, are long, flowing strokes. Your hands go under your partner's body *(back, neck, hips)* and you lift up as you draw your hands toward you. Your partner's body passively stretches as you perform your stroke.

It is an exquisite sensation to be lifted in this half stretch half stroke. As the body lets go of every tension, it feels almost weightless, if for but a moment.

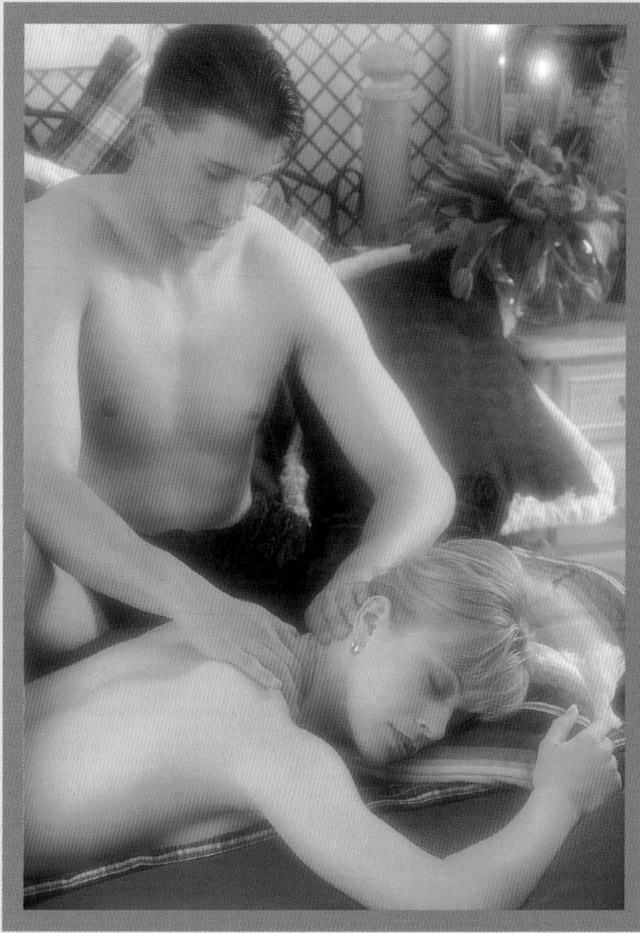

Kneading resembles short, lifting, and pulling strokes done in a rhythmic and continuous fashion to relax stubbornly tight muscles.

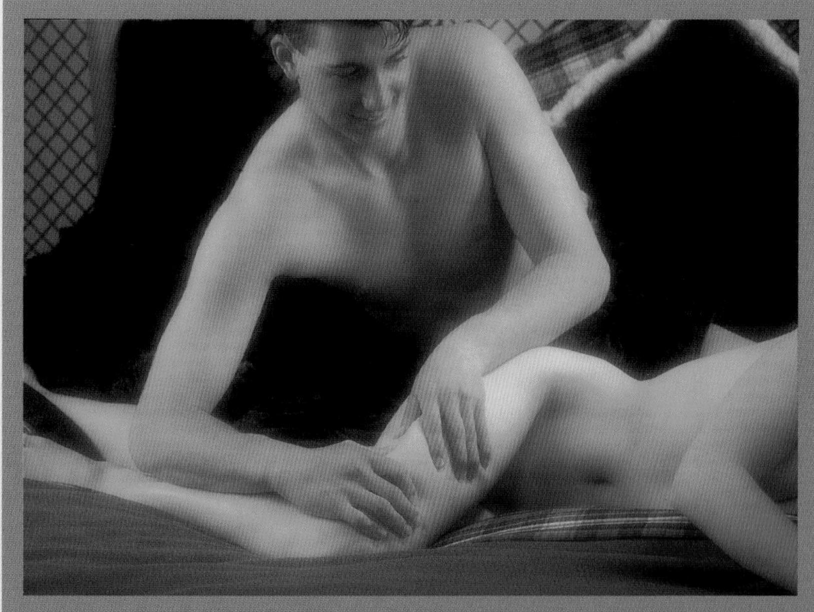

Although effleurage strokes are more sensual and erotic by nature, other massage strokes can be of great benefit and add to the overall mood in romantic massage. Many people hold muscle tension in their bodies; particularly in the neck, shoulders, and low back. As deeper, more aggressive strokes are used to break down this tension, we appreciate the relaxation and comfort they provide. The long, gliding strokes of effleurage, are a gentle and nurturing way to invite your partner to prepare for more invigorating Swedish massage strokes.

PETRISSAGE

Petrissage is short, grasping strokes to fleshy and muscular areas of the body to relax stubbornly tight muscles. As a result, fluids flow more easily through parts of the body normally congested by tension and fatigue. There are several variations of the petrissage stroke.

Kneading involves short lifting and pulling strokes in different directions that look very much like kneading bread dough. It is quite effective on arms and legs, buttocks, and any fleshy area.

You grasp the flesh with thumb and opposing fingers, pushing away from you with the thumb. Then, use your fingers to pull or roll the flesh back toward you. Both hands can perform this kneading action in unison, or alternating as one hand pushes away and the other pulls the flesh back.

Broad Kneading is sometimes called **Fulling**. It is a variation of petrissage performed by grasping the flesh and muscle with thumb and opposing fingers. Muscles are spread out in a flattening motion that makes the limb appear fuller than it really is.

This stroke is great on arms and legs. Both hands can grip and pull at the same time or in an alternating fashion.

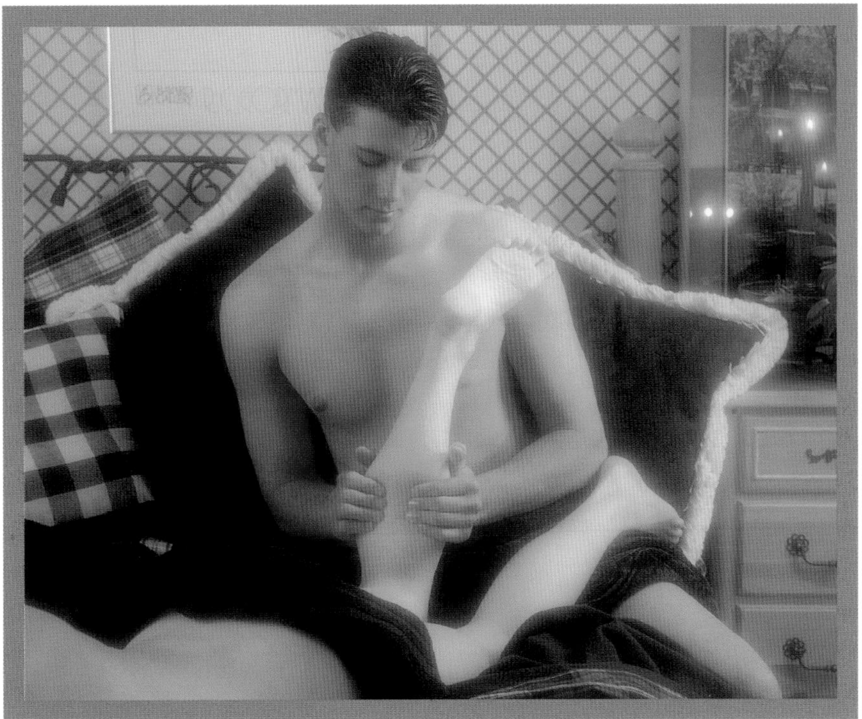

Broad Kneading or Fulling is a type of petrissage characterized by using the thumb and fingers to spread out and flatten fleshy areas on arms and legs.

Another variation is **Skin Rolling**. It is characterized by grasping a fleshy area with thumb and opposing fingers, lifting it up, and moving it in a rolling fashion.

Once the flesh is pinched up into a roll, the thumbs and fingers are inched along to continue to move the roll onward. The same section of flesh is not carried on past its normal space, but the fingers inch ahead gathering new flesh as the thumbs allow excess flesh to slip back behind. The roll continues; new areas are worked as the stroke advances.

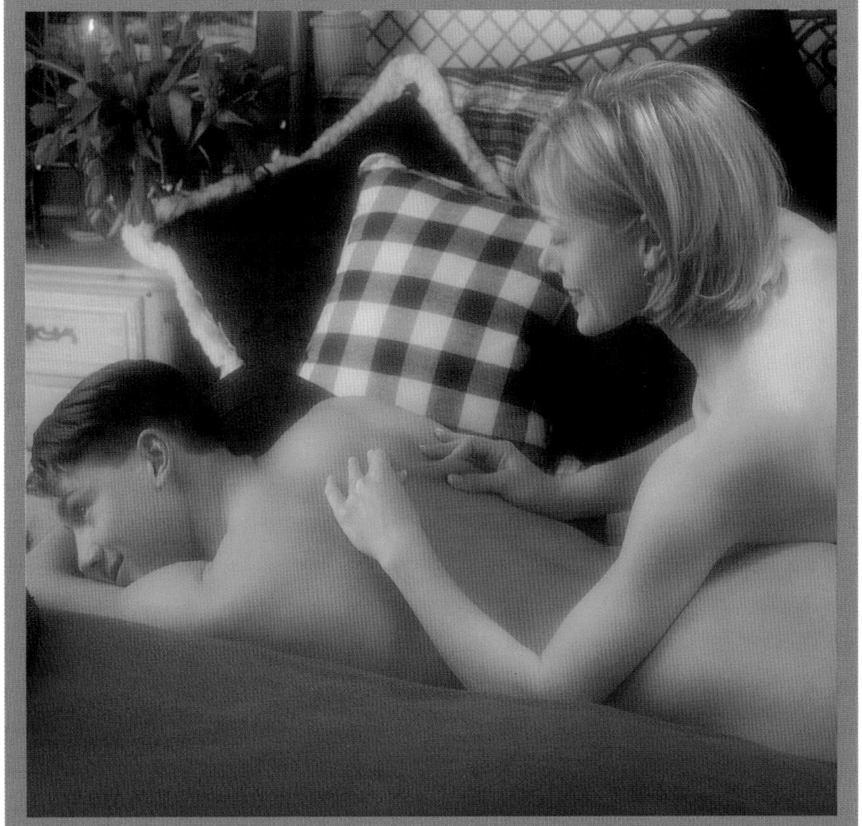

Skin Rolling gathers a section of flesh into a loose pinch. As the fingers inch along gathering new flesh, thumbs allow excess skin to drop back behind the area worked.

DEEP FRICTION

Friction is another Swedish massage stroke. It involves either dragging the hand over a body part, which creates heat from friction or taking superficial tissues and moving them over deeper layers, using medium to firm pressure, also creating a deep heating action. Friction strokes not only create heat through mildly aggressive friction movements, they also break down adhesions *(body tissues that abnormally adhere to one another)* and scar tissue.

Although friction strokes are not considered sensual, they provide a wondrous variety of pleasurable warming sensations.

Pressing or **Compression** is classified as a friction stroke; firm pressure is applied over muscle knots to break down chronically tense areas. You can use fingers, thumbs, knuckles, fists, or palms to apply pressure. Sometimes when the pressure is focused on a particularly tender area, the stroke can cause discomfort, if not pain. However, massage should not be a painful experience. In fact, hurting your partner is not conducive to romantic feelings.

Under normal situations, the most you should cause is mild discomfort. Always be aware of your partner's desires and try to satisfy them.

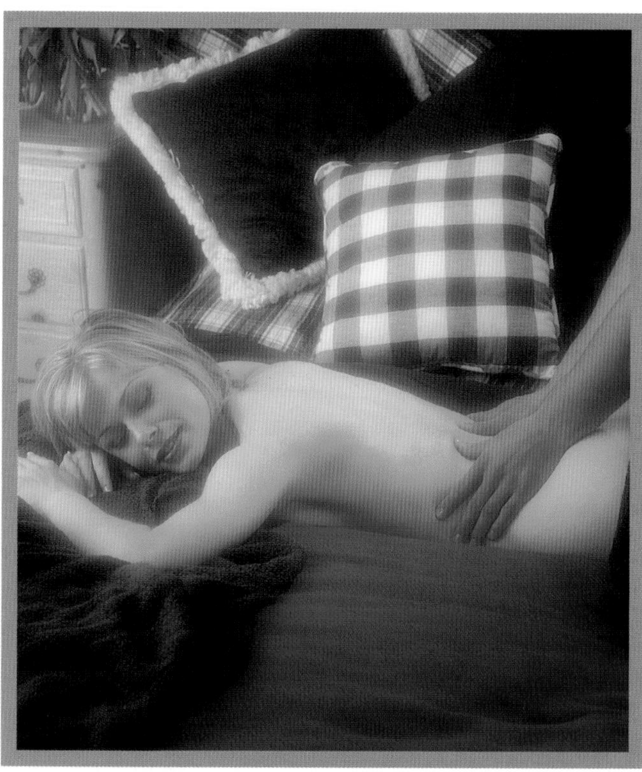

Thumb Compression is used to focus on tight muscles to help break down hard knots.

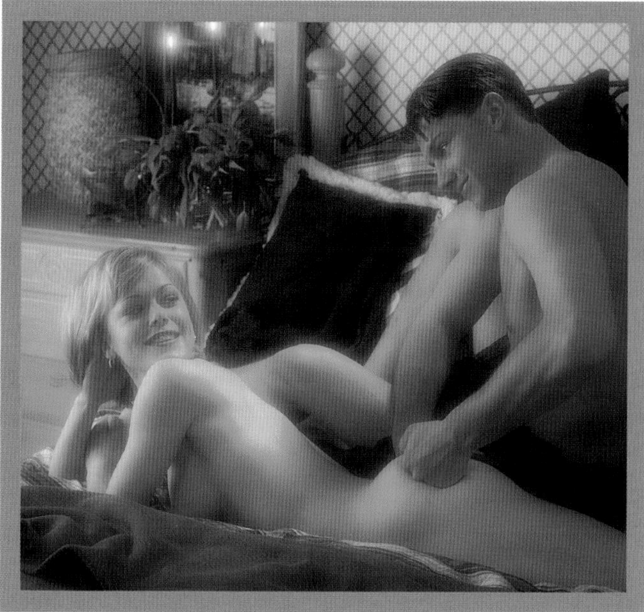

Pressing with fists helps to relieve tension in large, fleshy areas like the back or buttocks.

Purchase a fragrance ring that goes on top of a light bulb and place a few drops of fragrance specifically manufactured for fragrance rings or use your favorite essential oils to "scent" the mood.

- *For an outdoor mood try 5 drops: eucalyptus, myrtle, pine, rosemary, or spruce oil.*
- *Create a fragrant flower garden using 5 drops: benzoin, jasmine, bois de rose, or ylang-ylang oil.*
- *A citrus scent can be created by using 5 drops: lemon, lemongrass, lime, melissa, neroli, or orange oil.*

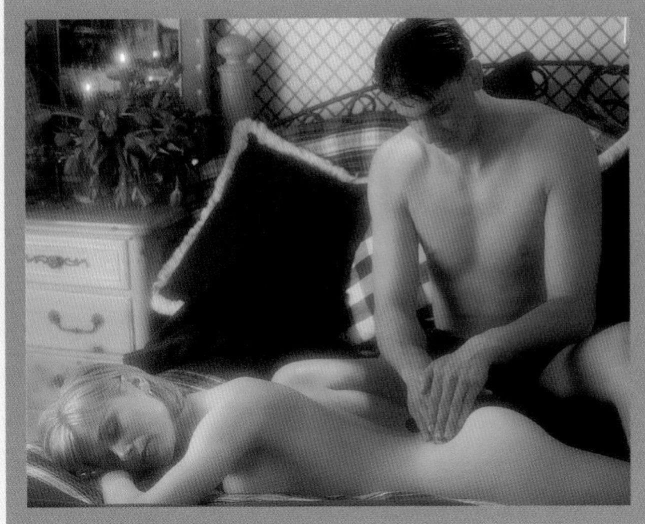

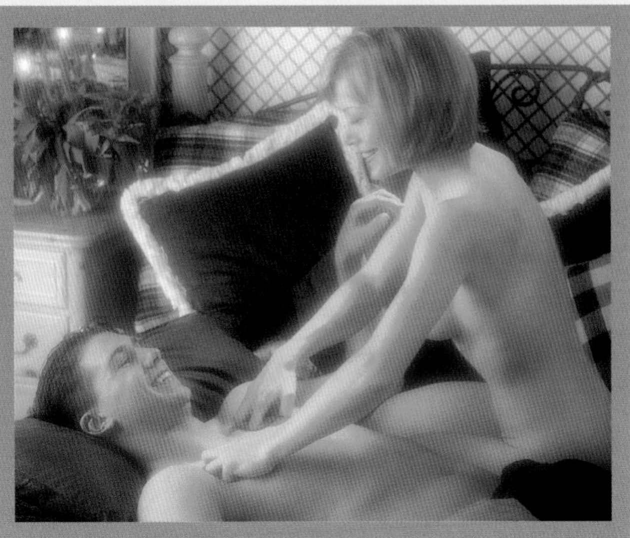

Circular Friction includes compression combined with circular movements which creates heat and can break down knots and adhesions.

This stroke can be executed using fingers, thumbs, knuckles, fists, or palms. Place moderately firm pressure over the area and make small circular motions. Slow circular motions are relaxing, while faster motions are stimulating to the body.

Knuckle Ironing is a blend of **deep effleurage** because the strokes are usually long with firm pressure, and **friction** because the deep knuckling causes heat and breaks down knots in muscles. The fingers are tucked under with the rest of the hand, open or in a loose fist. The wrist is usually straight to avoid undue stress or strain to wrist muscles and joint. Depending on the pressure applied, you may want to support the wrist joint by wrapping your free hand around it.

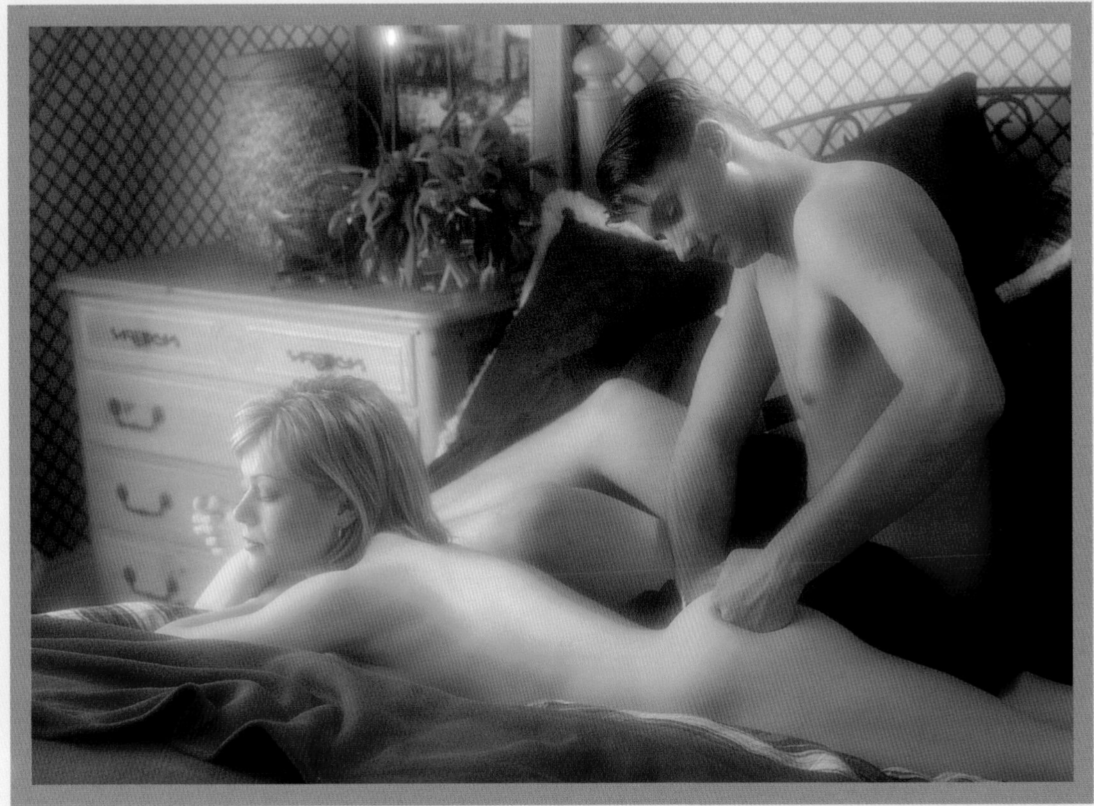

Wringing is a friction stroke where both hands grip an arm or leg and move in opposing directions. This stroke resembles wringing out a wet cloth. As flesh and muscles are pulled in opposing directions, friction causes heat and a break down of adhesions. Hands are side by side, and although the motion is slow, pressure is firm.

Cross Fiber Friction is similar to wringing, but hands are farther apart and less structured. This massage stroke goes across the muscle fiber orientation; for example, muscles run the length of the arm and the stroke moves across the fiber.

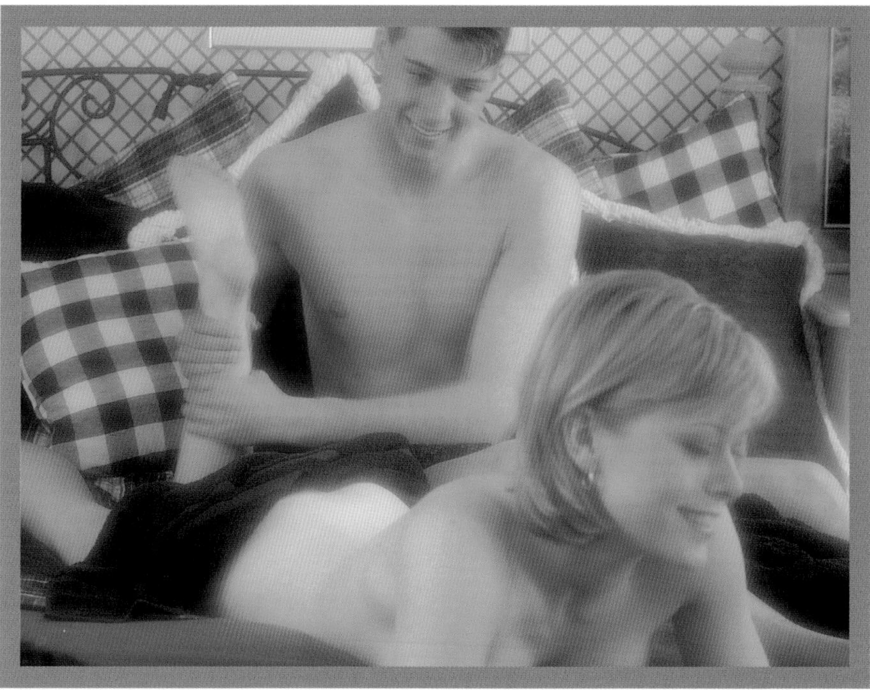

Wringing is a friction stroke where both hands grip a limb and move in opposing directions, like wringing out a wet cloth.

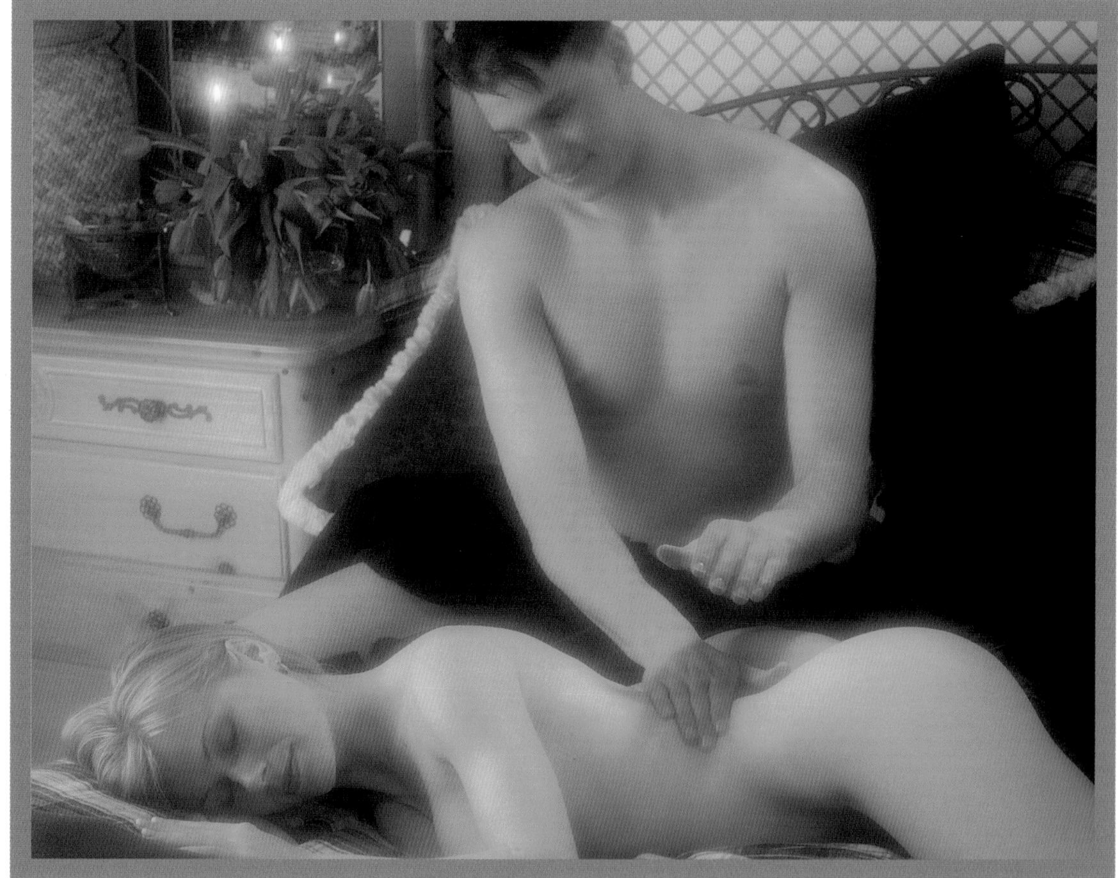

Cross Fiber Friction resembles a loose rendition of the wringing stroke, because the hands are not as close together.

VIBRATION

Vibration, the fourth of the five basic Swedish massage strokes is rhythmically shaking specific body parts to promote a deep and thorough relaxation of muscles. The premise behind this stroke is that the body naturally lets go of chronic tension while being shaken.

Rocking is gently swaying back and forth in a slow, rhythmic manner. The palms of the hands are placed on the area of the body to be rocked. Then, the heel of the palm pushes gently away and the fingers slowly pull back.

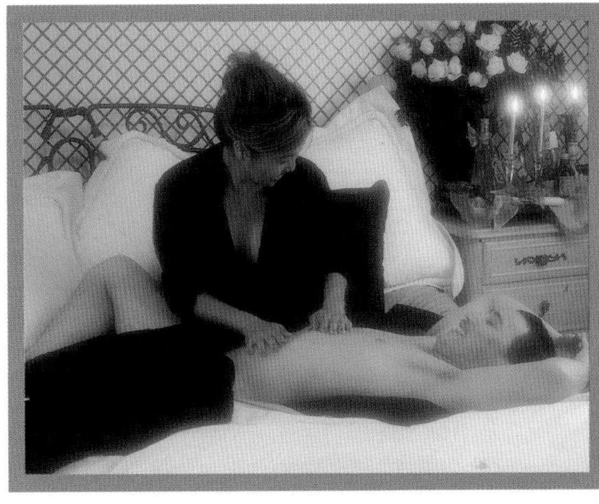

Rocking is gentle back and forth rhythmic movement.

Shaking is short, irregular to and fro movements. The palms of the hands are placed on the body area to be shaken and the heel of the palm pushes while the fingers draw back. However, the movements are small and irregular; as if to awaken your partner.

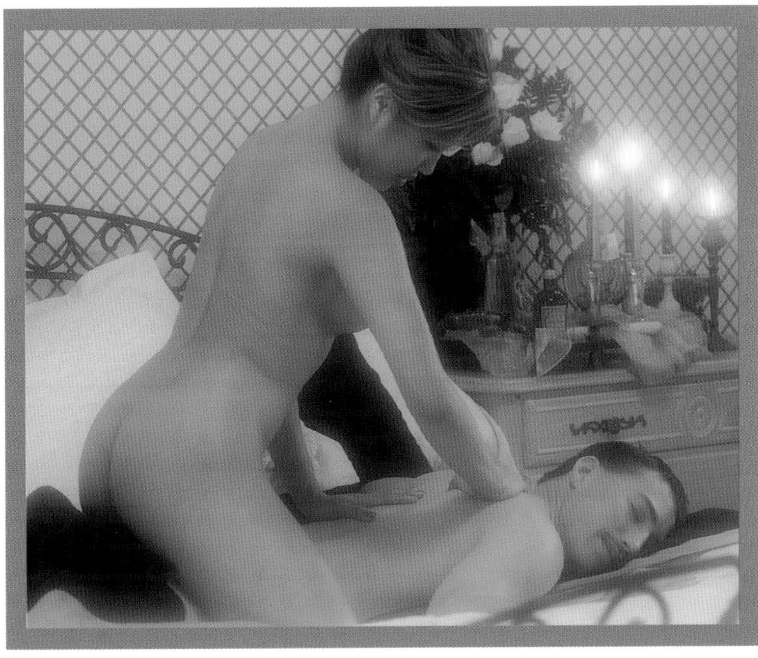

Shaking is short irregular to and fro movements.

Vibrating is moving back and forth in rapid rhythmic succession. It is highly stimulating and yet creates a deeply relaxing response after the stroke is complete.

Romantics:
- ♥ *are passionate, with a passion for life in general.*
- ♥ *"work at it" and "play at it," when scheming up a new romantic evening or event.*
- ♥ *are always dating and keeping romance fresh and alive.*
- ♥ *live in the moment, doing something romantic today and doing it with feeling!*

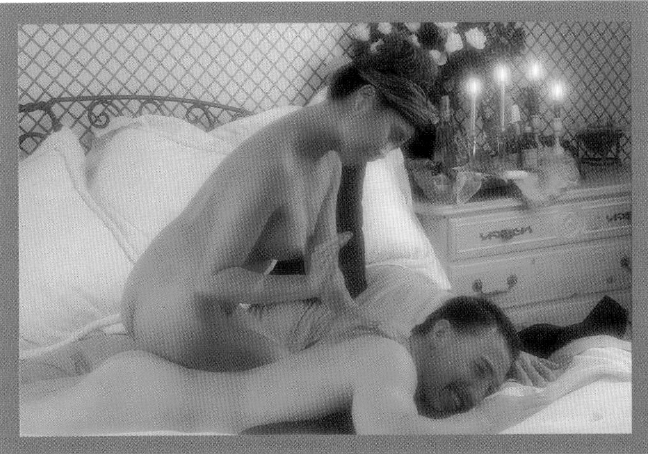

Vibrating is a rhythmic motion in rapid succession.

PERCUSSION/TAPOTEMENT

Percussion is the fifth and last category of Swedish massage strokes. It is a rhythmic striking of the skin. The effects of percussive strokes are highly stimulating. They bring blood to the surface of the skin quickly and aggressively move fluids to more areas of the body.

Depending on the force of the stroke, percussion can be very toning to muscles. That is, muscles that are struck, tighten up momentarily. This helps exercise muscles in instances of inactivity. It also forces lymph movement which increases the body's immune system response to help fight disease.

Lastly, percussive strokes help nourish and beautify skin as blood is forced to the surface. The striking action and increased blood flow help loosen fatty deposits and increase their metabolism by the body.

Percussive strokes are not part of the normal repertoire of strokes in a relaxing or romantic massage, but variety is the spice of life. If your partner enjoys them, playful slaps and taps can be used to liven and arouse. Just be certain that your partner is agreeable to these particular massage strokes.

Tapping is where the fingertips or pads are used to lightly tap the skin. All fingers can hit simultaneously or at different times to create a pitter patter effect. This "raindrops" effect is excellent on the face, scalp, and any erogenous zones of the body.

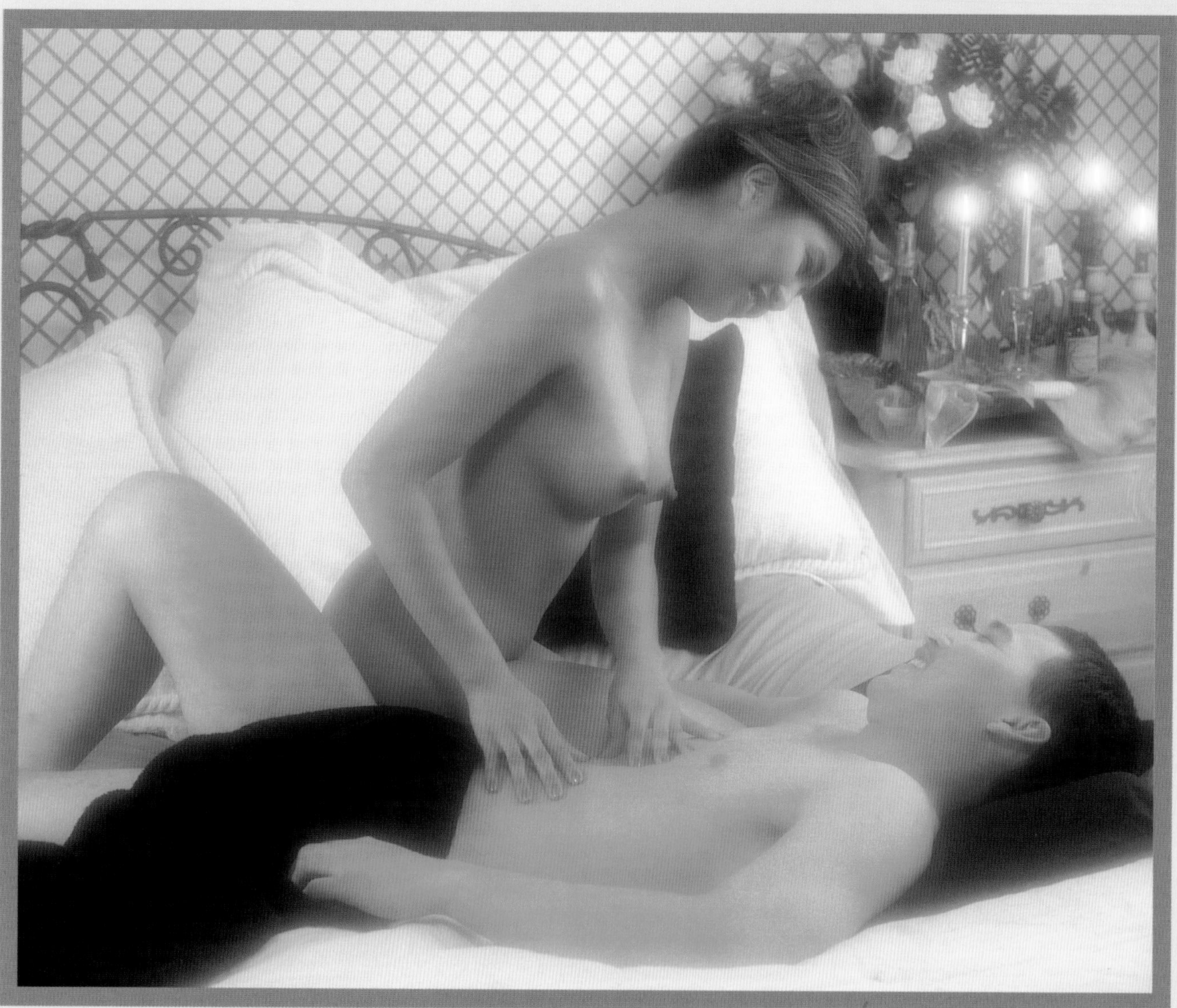

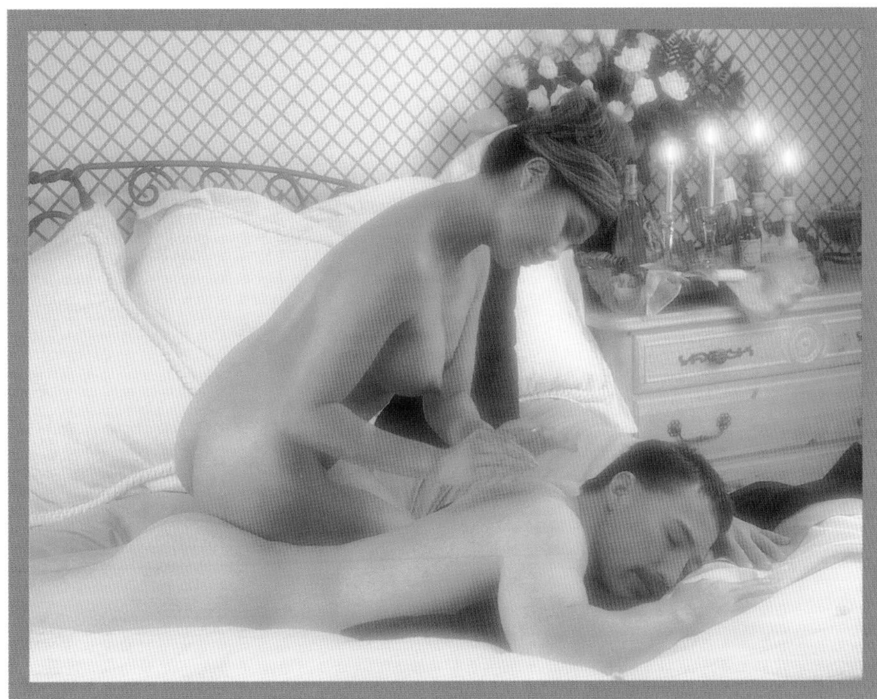

Cupping is not as highly stimulating as slapping, but, it is safe to use even over bony areas.

Playful slaps offer some spice to your romantic massage to liven and arouse.

Cupping is similar to slapping with one exception — the hand is shaped concavely (like a cup) with fingers and thumb together. It is not as highly stimulating as slapping, but it runs a close second to hacking and beating. It is safe to use over bony and normally sensitive areas of the body.

Slapping occurs when the entire hand (palm and fingers) in a relaxed state, strikes the skin. The effect to the body depends on the force of the stroke. It is highly stimulating to skin and nerves. (You may need to prepare your partner because slapping and cupping may produce a startling sound.)

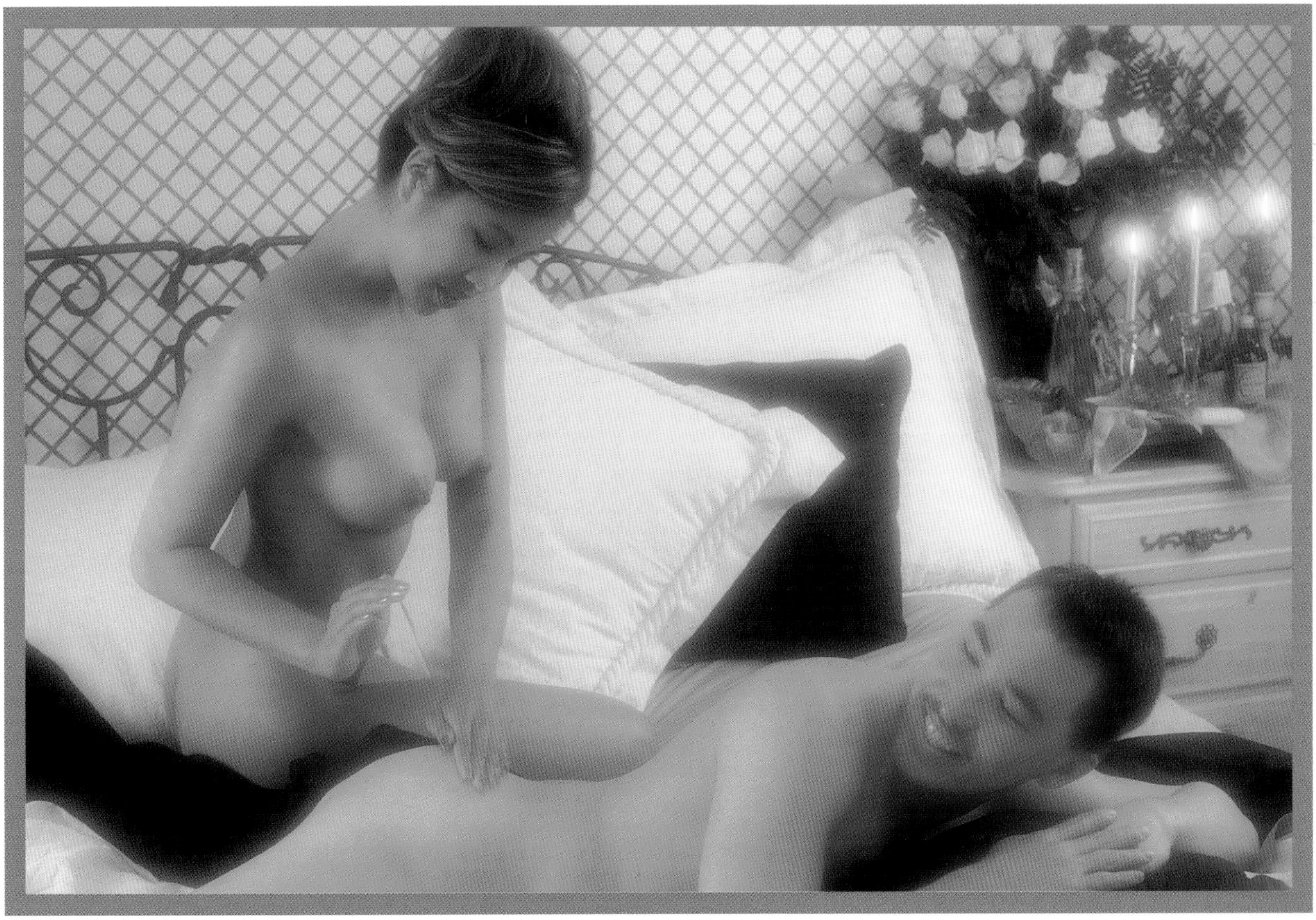

Beating or **Pummeling** is rapid striking of skin with the edge or flat of a clenched fist. This stroke should be done only over fleshy or muscular regions like the thighs or buttocks because of its aggressiveness. Avoid the low back (kidney punch), bony, or tender areas.

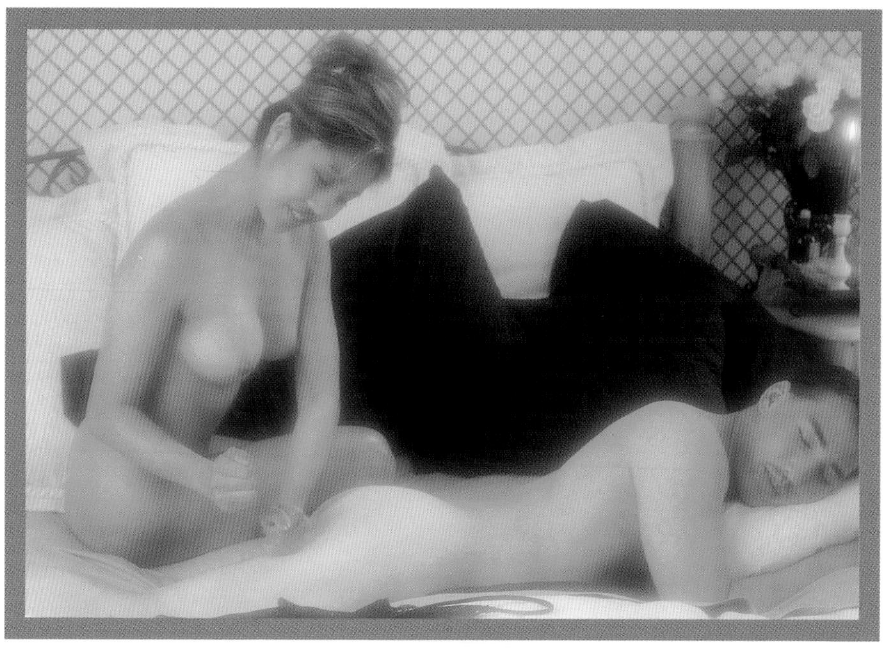

Pummeling is an aggressive stroke and should be avoided over the low back, bony areas, and any sensitive place.

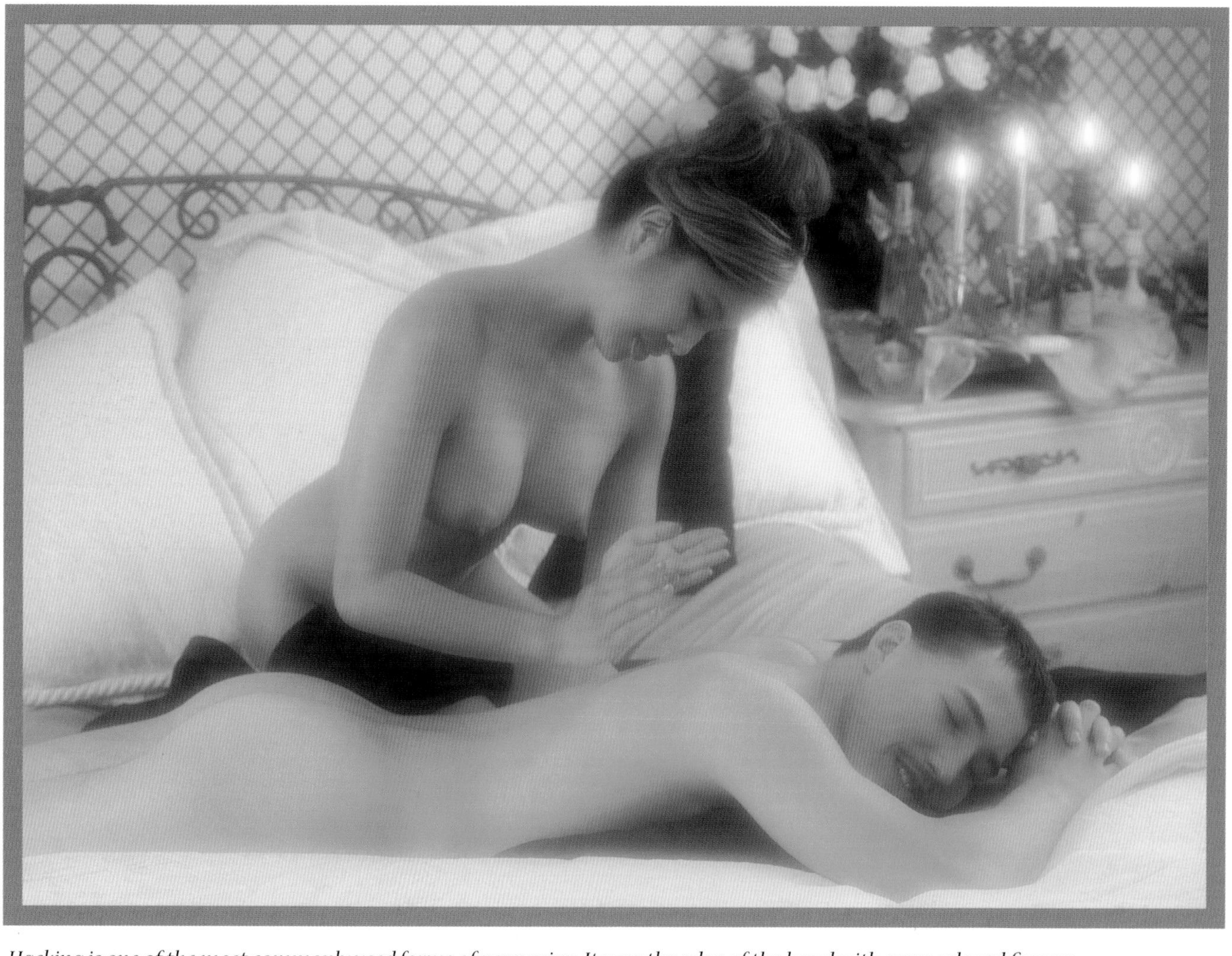

Hacking is similar to pummeling. The edge of the hand is used for the stroke, but fingers are open and relaxed not clenched in a fist. Avoid this stroke on bony areas. This stroke is highly stimulating.

Hacking is one of the most commonly used forms of percussion. It uses the edge of the hand with open, relaxed fingers.

Two percussive strokes that are popular in Europe are plucking and whipping.

Plucking is the grasping of an amount of flesh with the thumb and opposing fingers, pulling it up rapidly, and letting it slip through the grasp. It is not as toning as other forms of percussion, but it definitely stimulates skin and nerves.

Whipping is when the hands rotate rapidly at the wrist like whipping cream using a spoon. The fingers are held together and are used to execute the stroke. It is not a strongly forceful stroke, but again it is stimulating to skin and nerves.

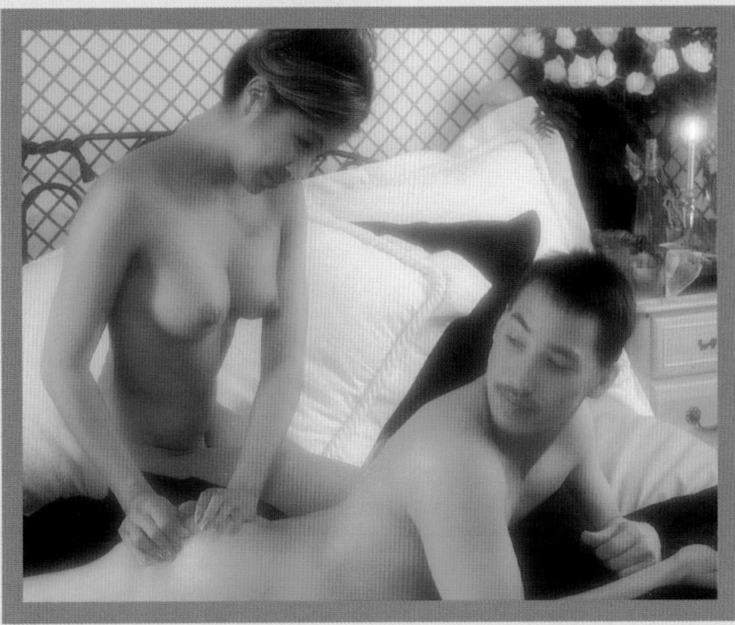

Plucking is made by grasping flesh with thumb and opposing fingers, pulling up rapidly and letting go.

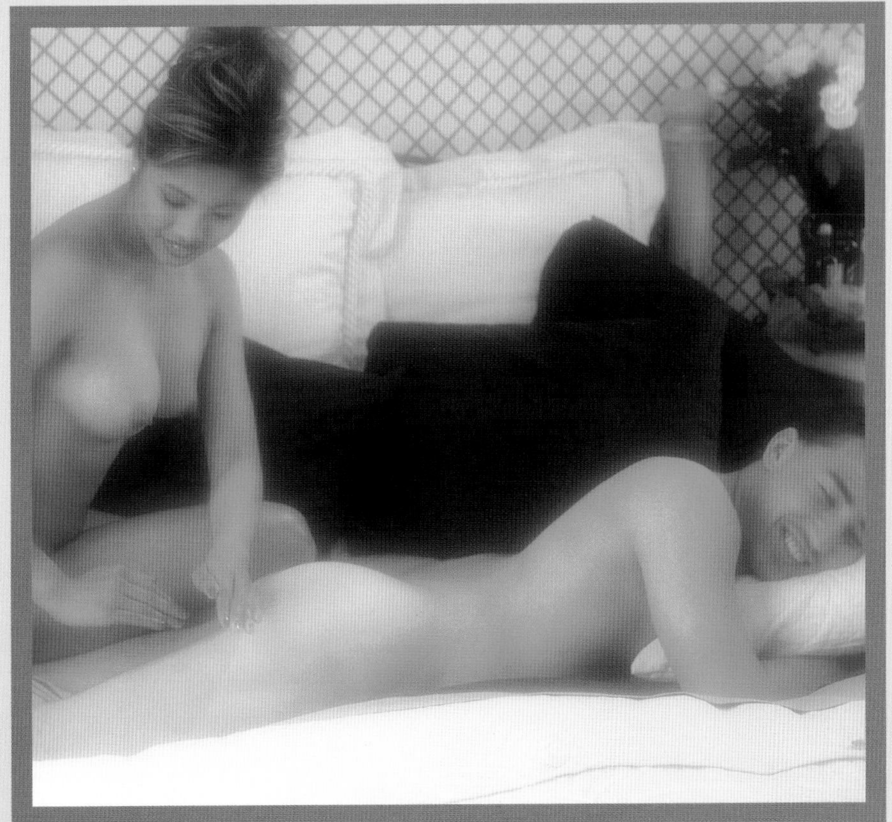

Whipping is literally "all in the wrist." Rotate the wrist rapidly and whip the skin lightly with your fingers.

Variety — the Spice of Life

Remember, using one stroke for too long can cause your partner to lose the sensual response the massage is trying to evoke. Long flowing strokes can be done up to ten times each, petrissage for several minutes, friction for a minute or two, and vibration or percussion long enough for the effects to be felt.

Use your imagination. You know what your lover likes and wants. If you don't know, ask. Make it sensually pleasurable. Your goal may not be seductive foreplay that leads to sex. It may be time to just tease and explore.

You know what your lover wants. Use your imagination when making a massage sensually pleasurable and seductive.

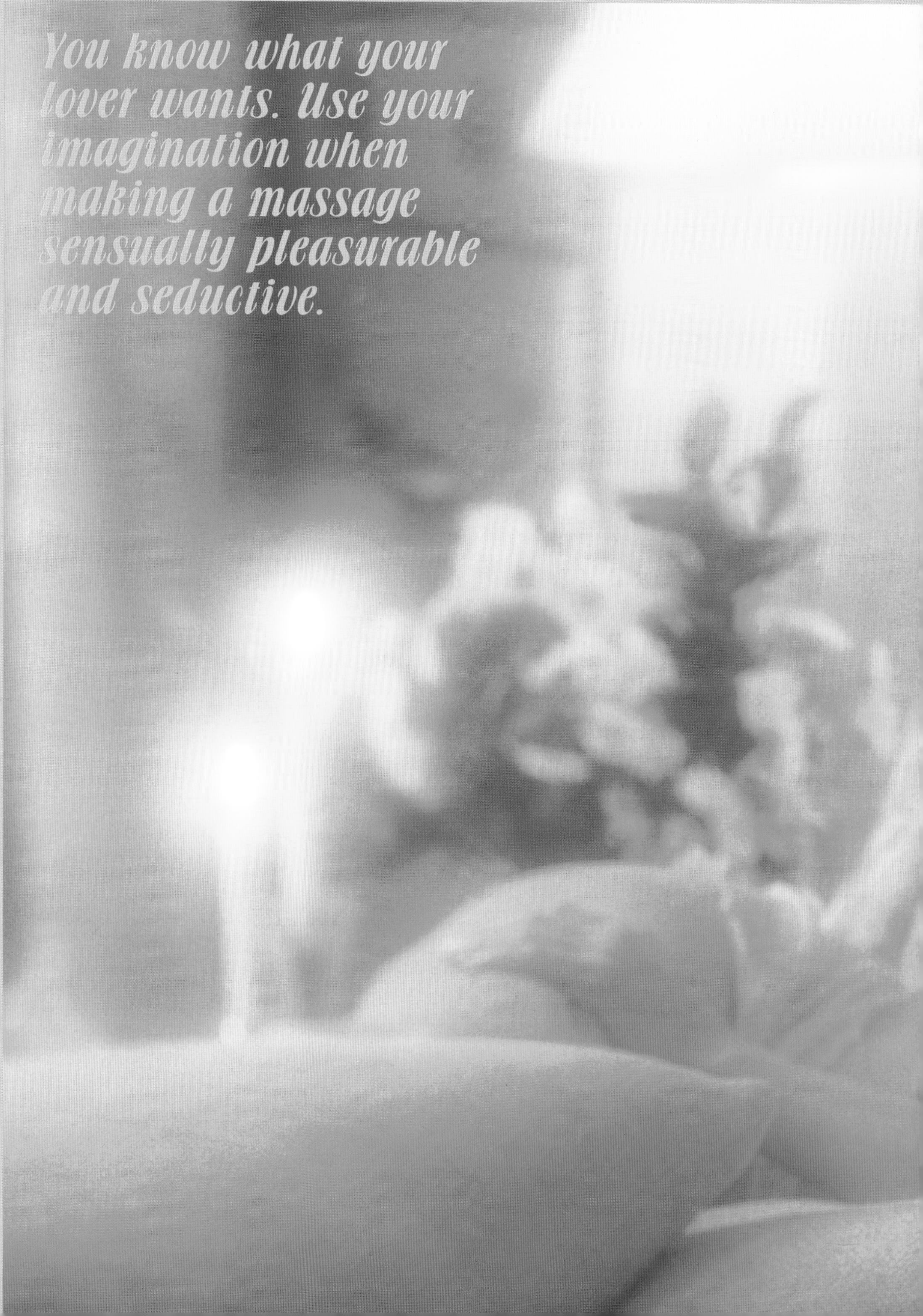

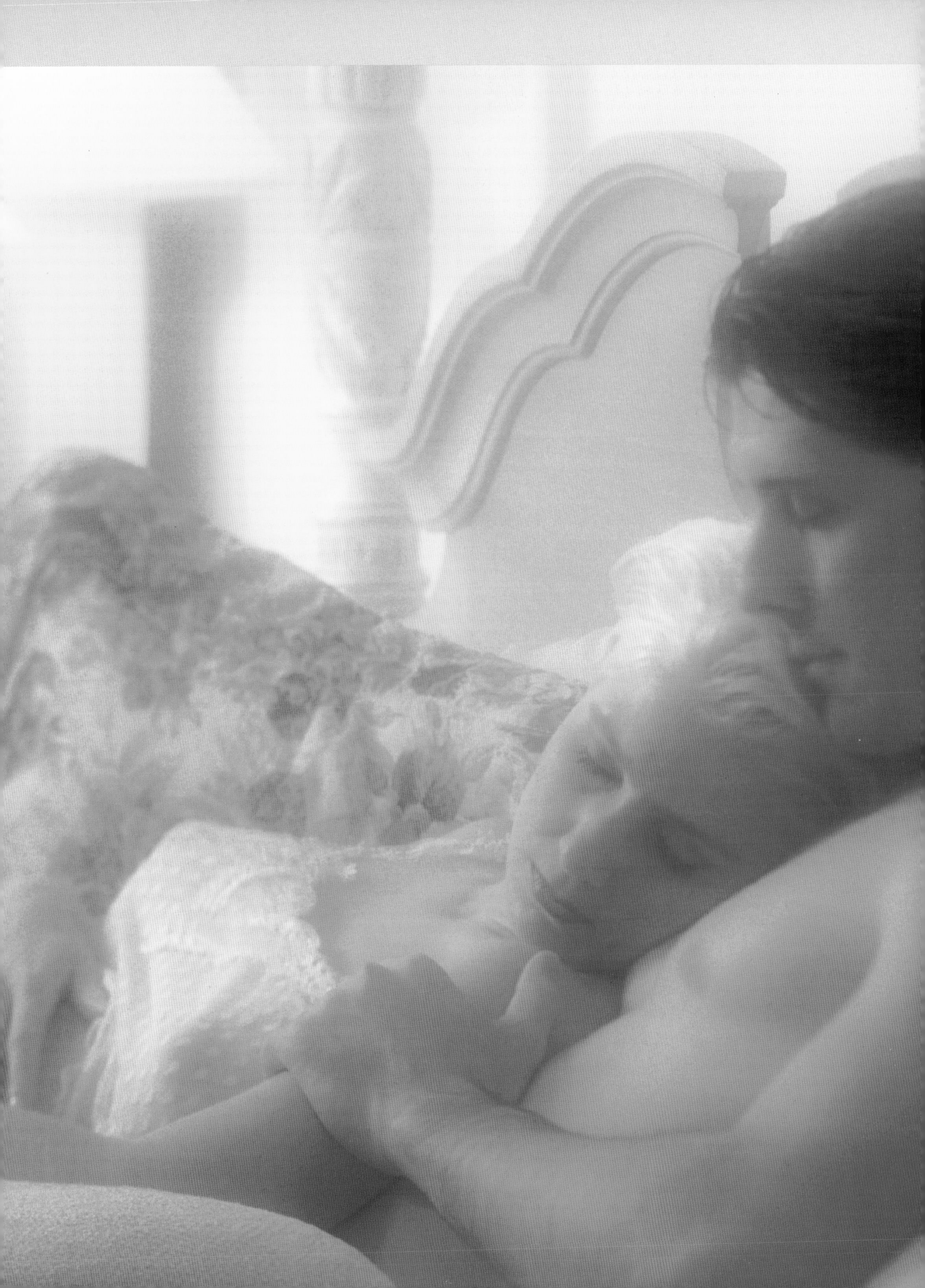

chapter five

Tender Beginnings

Sensual, erotic, romantic massage incorporates not only the relaxation strokes of effleurage, but the more aggressive strokes of petrissage, friction, vibration and tapotement. The soft strokes that release tension can be followed by strokes of deep pressure that penetrate muscles. Blend this with light and tender caresses that tantalize and arouse romantic feelings.

While relaxing your lover, your massage should stimulate and heighten the senses through touch and movement. Play, using your entire body to make contact. Brush gently, sense the change in their breathing that speaks of excitement. Tease and leave, in your touch, the promise of more to come.

Touch. Explore. Enjoy the pleasure both of you receive from each new discovery as your hands linger with each stroke. Allow the different massage strokes to blend into a flow of sensuous touches and tickles.

The sensations of pleasure become so intense for you both that you can anticipate each other's needs and responses as the massage progresses. It becomes an electrifying experience during this romantic time together.

Our bodies have a bio-energy field called an aura. The aura is enhanced and energized as you begin to massage your lover. With each and every touch, every stroke, your lover's body becomes sensitized.

It is logical that if your partner's body has an invisible energy field that is stimulated when massaged; you have an energy field too. Your aura connects to their aura even before the massage begins. And, as you touch, the "electricity," the chemistry, between you increases in intensity. The fire within grows at a phenomenal rate given the proper stimuli, —touches and tickles, probes and prods, delicate stroking, and sensitive caresses. That is romantic massage!

Whether you spend an hour or an evening, if you rub the neck and shoulders or give a full body massage, whether you just explore and enjoy or incorporate massage as a prelude to sex, the choice is yours. You are about to discover a wondrous variety of emotions.

This is not a fixed recipe of moves and maneuvers guaranteed to arouse the person you touch. But between sensitive, consenting lovers, it opens the possibilities of pleasuring like no other.

What is your partner really saying?

- ♥ *Listen for the meaning behind the words. Tune in to your partner and listen for the emotional content, not just the words. We do not always say what we really mean.*
- ♥ *Look for the non-verbal cues. Read the subtle body signals that your partner uses. Being able to read your partner's body language will help develop a better and more loving relationship.*

Neck & Shoulder Sequence

1 Begin by letting your partner sit or kneel on the bed. You and your partner do not need to have your clothes off at this time. You may simply want to allow the straps to fall off the shoulder of your partner's teddy or neglige.

As you begin the massage, contact is very important. It sets the mood for what is to come later. Rest your hands on your partner's shoulders, one hand on either side of the base of the neck. No massage oil is needed at this time.

Feel the muscles under your hands. The back, shoulders, neck, and head are among the most common areas to retain muscle tension in the body. The warmth of your hands resting on your lover's shoulders can help melt away unwanted aches and pains.

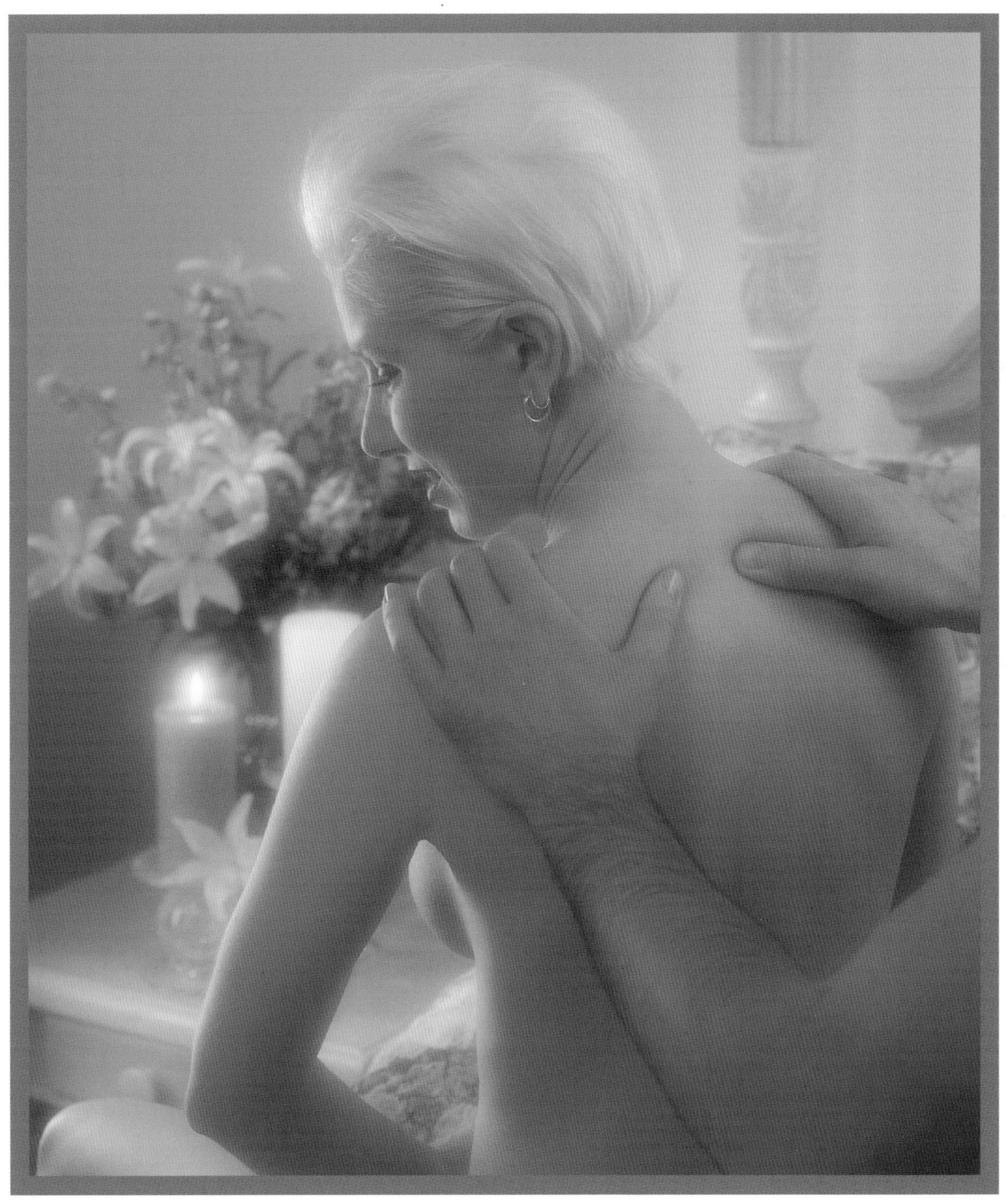

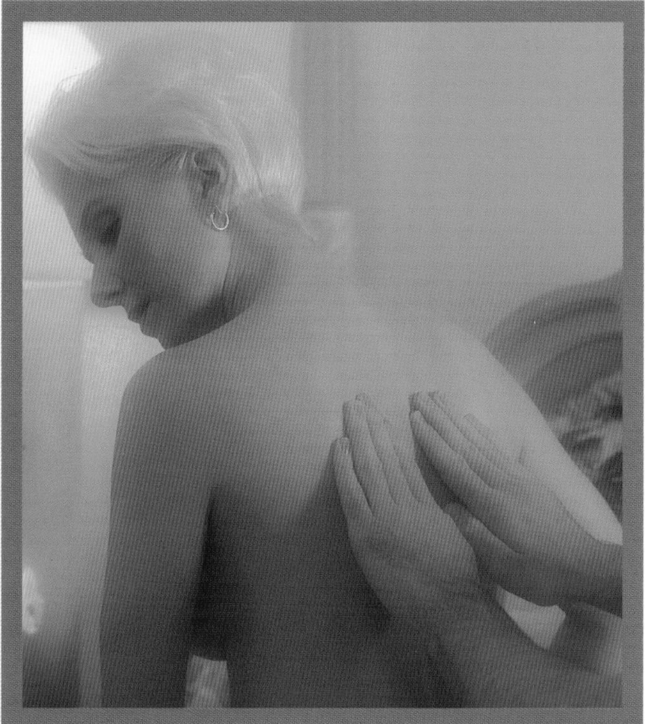

2 Let your hands slide down between the shoulder blades. Then, glide your hands up on either side of the spine until they reach the top of the shoulders. From there, allow your hands to flow out to the ends of the shoulders and down the arms. Repeat several times.

3 During the last glide to the top of your partner's shoulders, rest your hands at the top on either side of the base of the neck. Squeeze the shoulder muscles with the heel of your hand and opposing fingers. Move outward about an inch and squeeze again. Do this to the ends of the shoulders and down the arms to just above the elbow. Repeat several times.

3a Bring your hands to the top of the shoulders. This time use your thumb to make little circles half way down the back on either side of the spine, an inch or two out from the spine. Your thumb pressure activates oriental acupoints good for the respiratory and circulatory systems. Repeat several times.

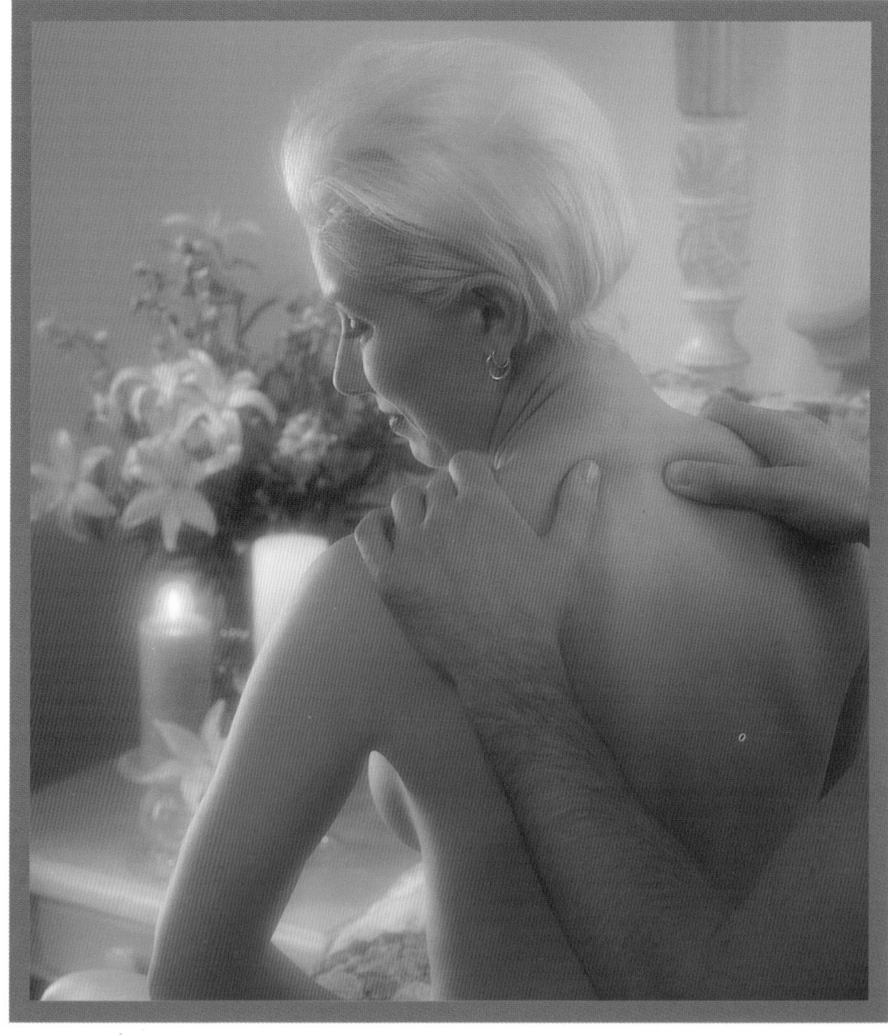

Keep the romance alive:
- ♥ *Spread fresh rose petals on pillows and sheets.*
- ♥ *Write or copy a love poem on scented stationery or parchment and leave it on your lover's pillow.*
- ♥ *When is the last time you said, "I love you."*
- ♥ *Kidnap your lover for a romantic evening or a romantic weekend.*

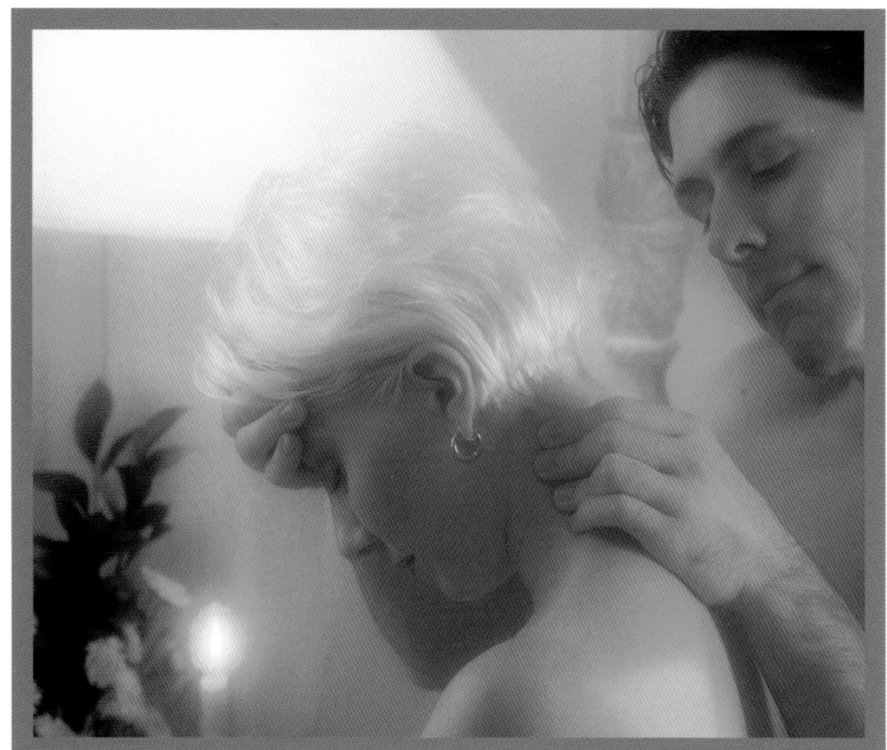

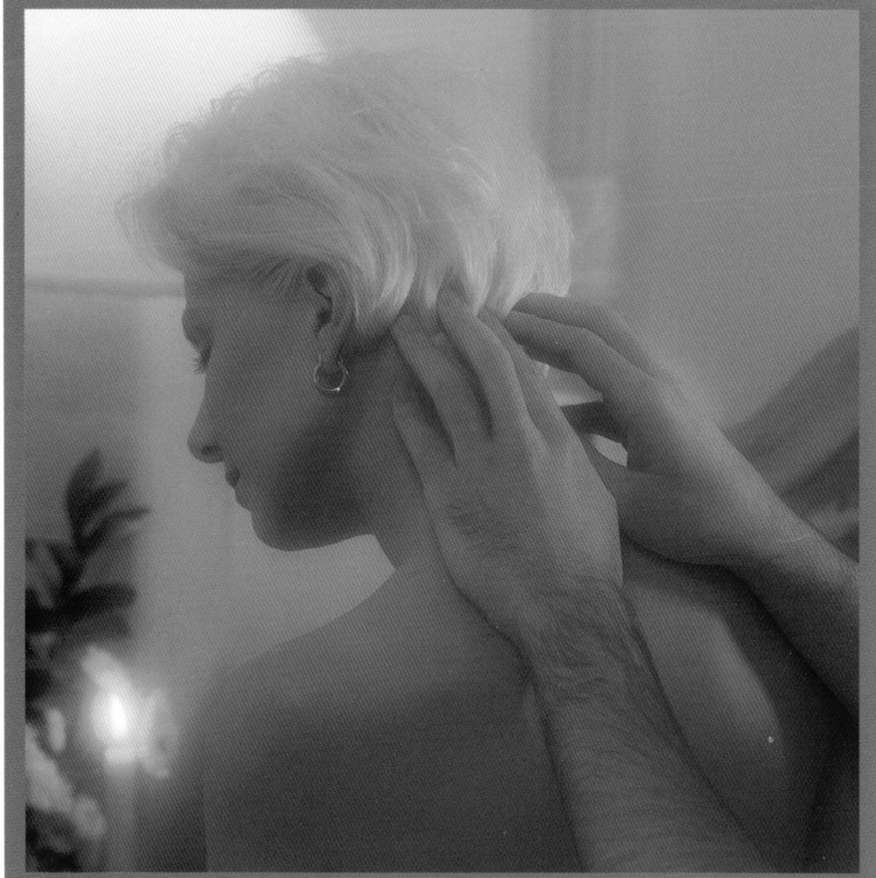

Massaging the skull can relieve tension headaches and pain associated with staring at computer screens, one of the various types of repetitive stress.

4 While leaving one hand on your partner's back, move to one side. Support their head with your free hand; encourage relaxation and take the weight of their head in your hand. Massage the neck by using gentle compression with your thumb and opposing fingers. Begin at the base of the neck and squeeze. Move up an inch or two and squeeze again. Repeat all the way up the neck. You may also add some circular friction with this stroke from the base, all the way up the back of the neck. Repeat several times. As you find tension, spend a little extra time and apply a little additional pressure to work it out.

5 Tilt your partner's head upright for this next move. Take your thumb and press up and into the muscles just beneath the ridge all along the base of the skull. Use slow and gentle pressure when working at the base of the skull if your partner experiences any pain.

How sweet the love
that meets return,
How dear the sunny smile,
Lighting up eyes
that on us burn
With love lights
all the while.
How soft the sigh
breathed forth by lips
That speak love's tender vow,
Cheering the heart
as sunlight tips
The hills with golden glow.
Tracy Gill

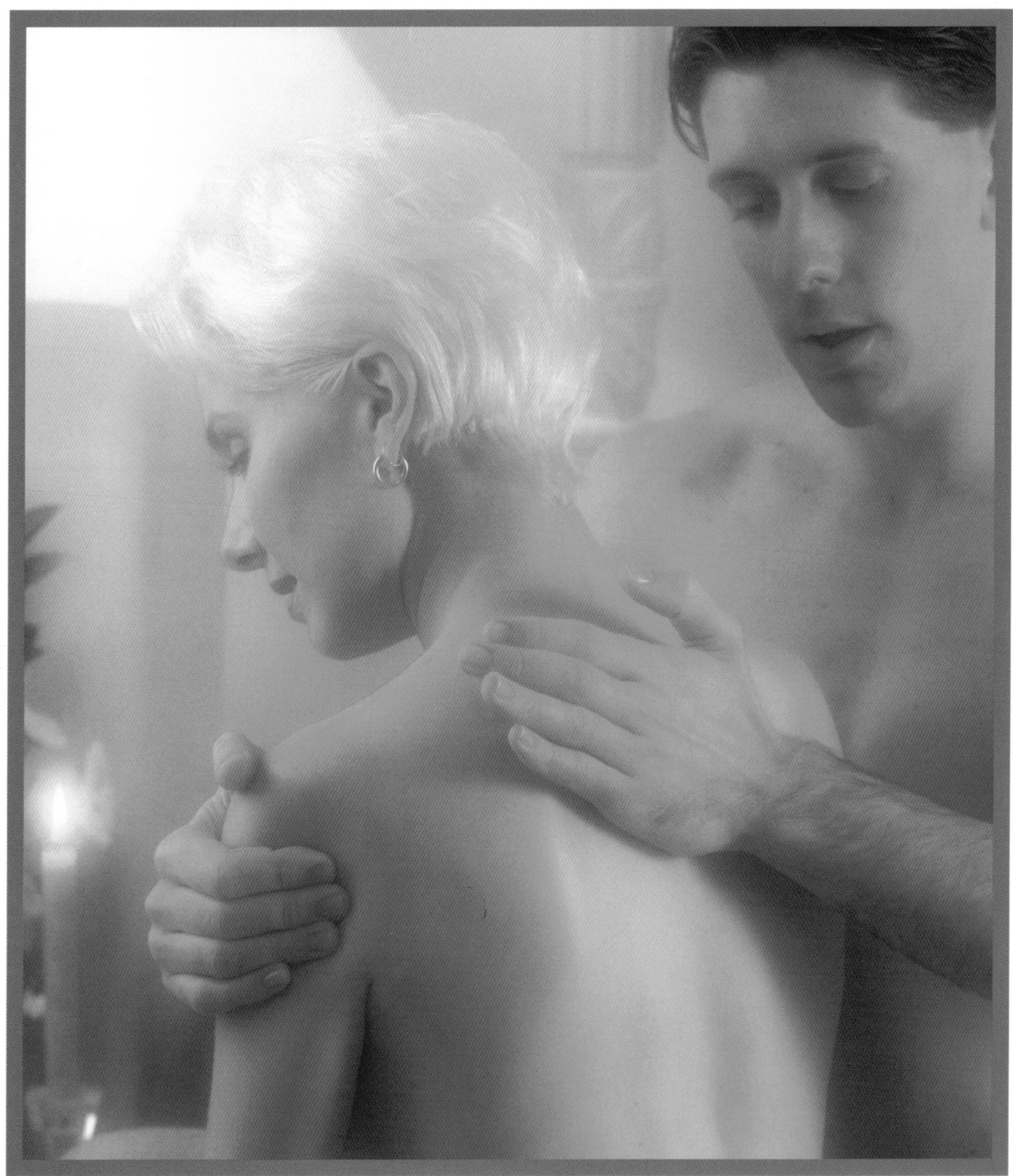

6 Using the heel of your hand, apply firm pressure, and make medium circles from between the shoulder blades and all the way down the back on both sides of the spine. Some spinal muscles may be quite tense. Vary your pressure to help relax these muscles. Repeat this sequence on each side of the spine several times.

Kiss every square inch of your lover's body
S-L-O-W-L-Y

Addressing the Back

If you want to relax the entire body, massage the back. Whether we stand or sit, bend or twist, back muscles are used; become fatigued, and are stressed by physical pressure placed on the spine.

Tight spinal muscles place undue pressure on the intervertebral discs, which cushion the vertebra in the spine. This, in turn, places pressure on the spinal nerves that are close to these discs. The pressure on the nerves can cause pain or numbness. By relaxing back muscles with massage, the spine lengthens, taking pressure off the back.

Spinal nerves feed the entire body, so virtually every stroke you perform on the back will affect the rest of the body. Each major organ in your partner's body will benefit from the effects of your massage.

1 Have your partner lie face down and then sit, or kneel next to your partner, or straddle them. You will want to anoint your partner's back with oil. Pour ½–1 teaspoon of warmed oil into the palm of your hand. Rub your hands together. Begin with some long light strokes up the back to spread the oil. Your hands will drag with too little oil. Too much oil will cause slipping and sliding. You will want to use just the right amount of oil to lubricate and still allow for friction strokes.

1a When you need additional oil, maintain body contact with one hand, drawing it slowly and lightly across the back on a return stroke. Pour additional oil onto the back of the hand, and use your other hand to apply oil to the back. In this way, your partner does not feel a break in the massage stroke and can continue to relax.

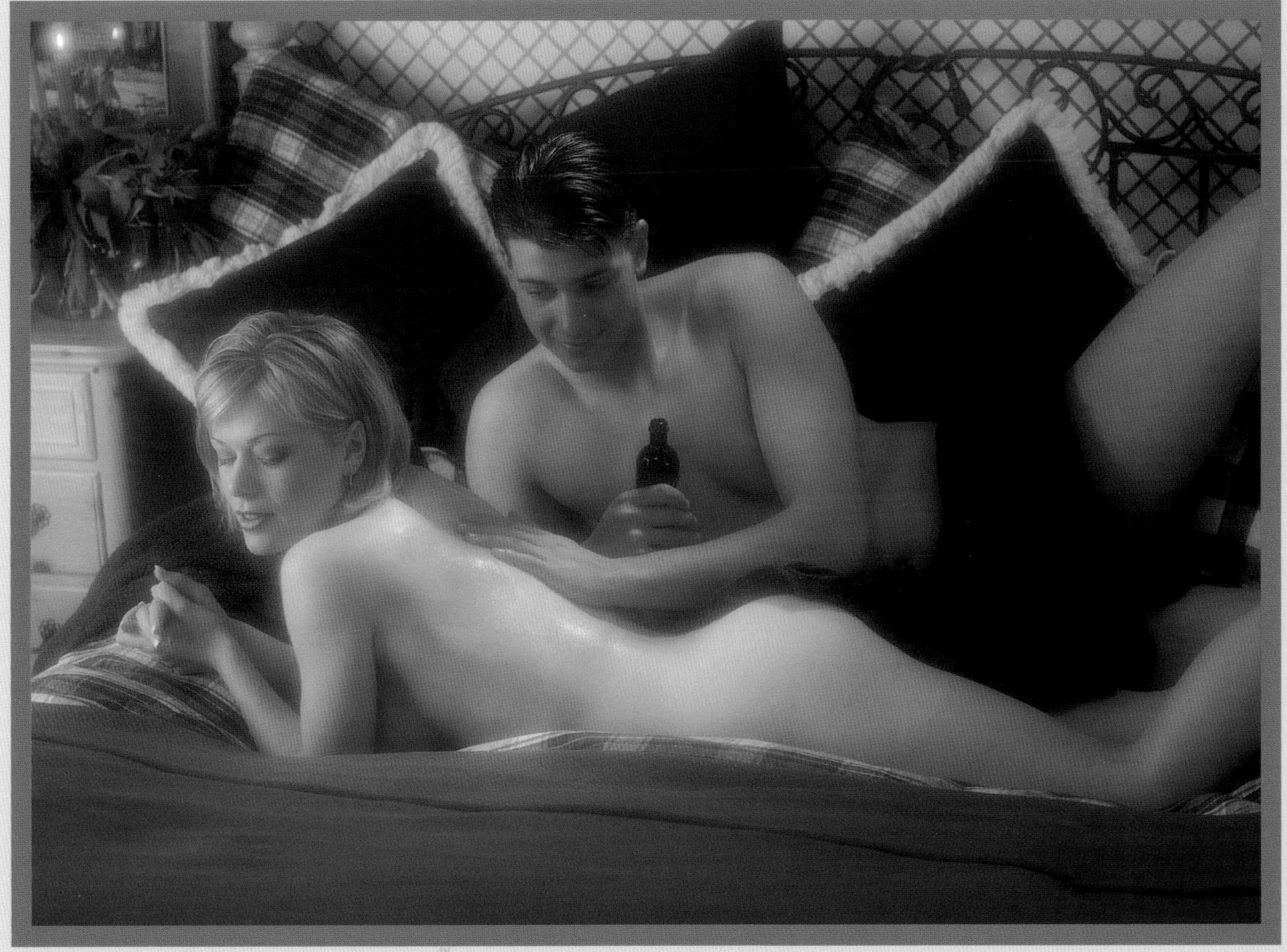

2 Begin to soothe the back muscles by using light to medium effleurage up the back on each side of the spine. Start the stroke just above the buttocks. Continue up the back to the top of the shoulders. Then, sweep your hands out over the ends of the shoulders, and down the side of the back. As your hands reach the hips, go up and over to repeat the stroke. Be certain your hands are flat, relaxed, and in contact with your partner's back. Let them glide over the soft contours of the shoulders, back, hips, and buttocks. Linger, ever so slightly, where the gluteal fold begins. This is an arousal point.

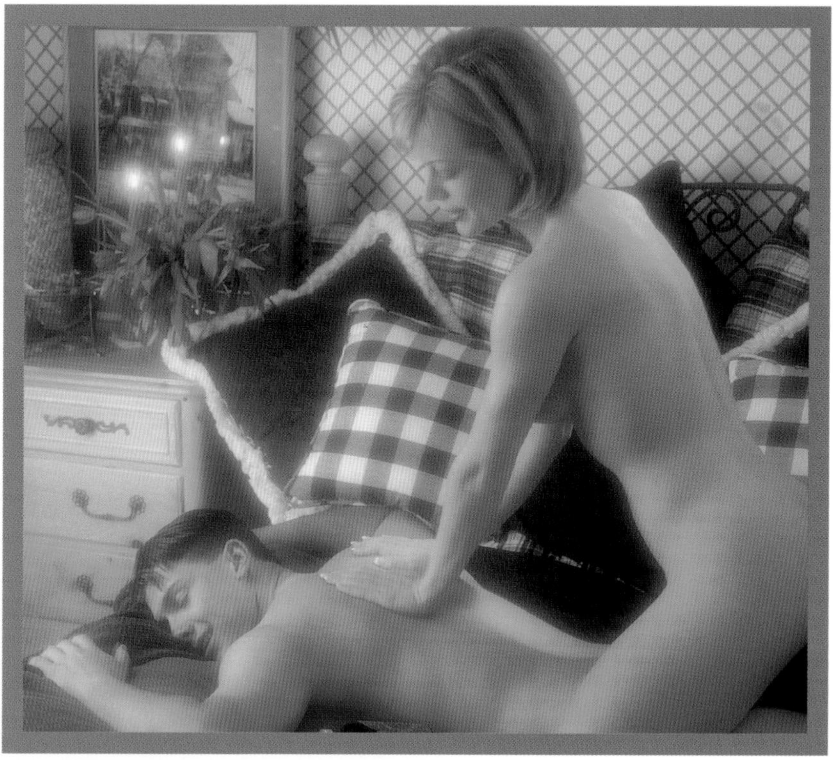

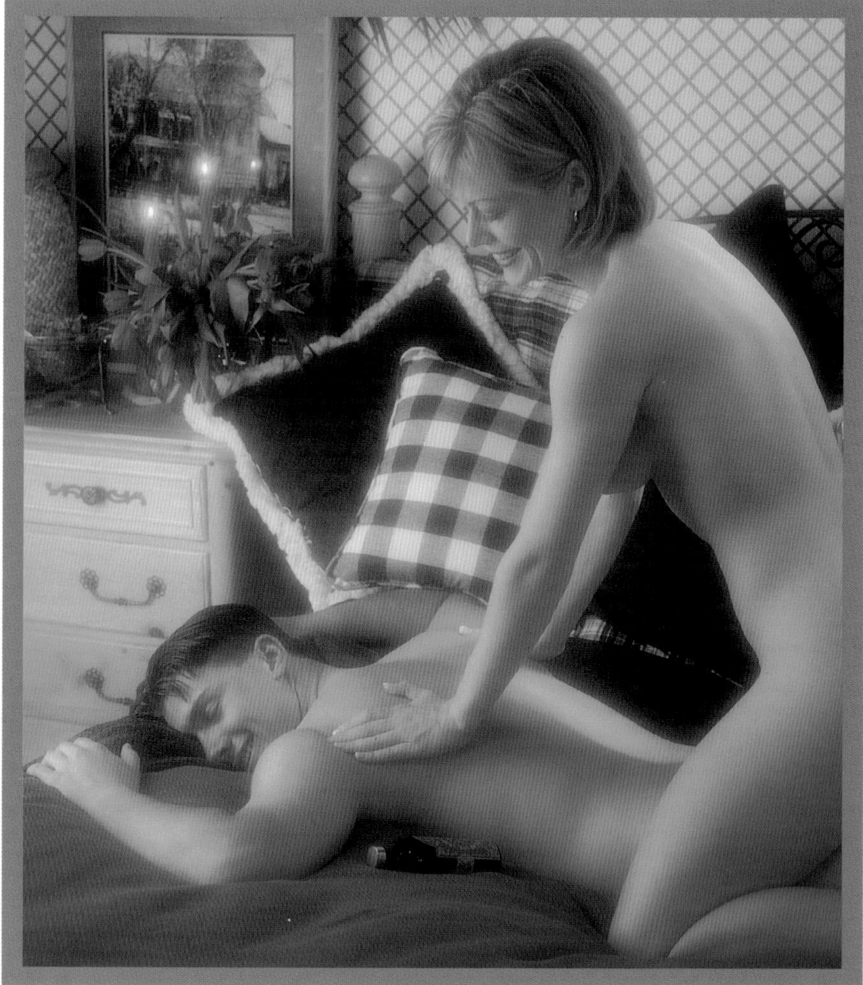

2a Continue this long back stroke. Correspond each stroke with your partner's breath. Push on the exhale, return stroke with the inhale. With each successive stroke up the back, slightly increase pressure to the muscles. The return stroke should always be lighter than your main stroke. Lean into the strokes to create more pressure. Apply more pressure with your fingertips. You will be able to tell when your partner's muscles relax and when to go deeper. You can ask if your pressure is sufficient, but keep conversation to a minimum. This should be a time of quiet and repose. As you continue this stroke, you may want to include long flowing massage strokes to the buttocks. Your partner can enjoy these long strokes for several minutes, if desired.

3 Now, use petrissage or short, grasping strokes on the back. Begin at the shoulders. This stroke always feels great, because of all of the stress and tension held in the shoulder muscles. Remember to work slowly. Grasp the thick shoulder muscle — trapezius — between your thumb and fingers. Squeeze and tease as you work the muscles, like kneading bread dough. Your lover will respond quickly by relaxing and enjoying your touch. Repeat this stroke to the shoulders as many as ten times on each side.

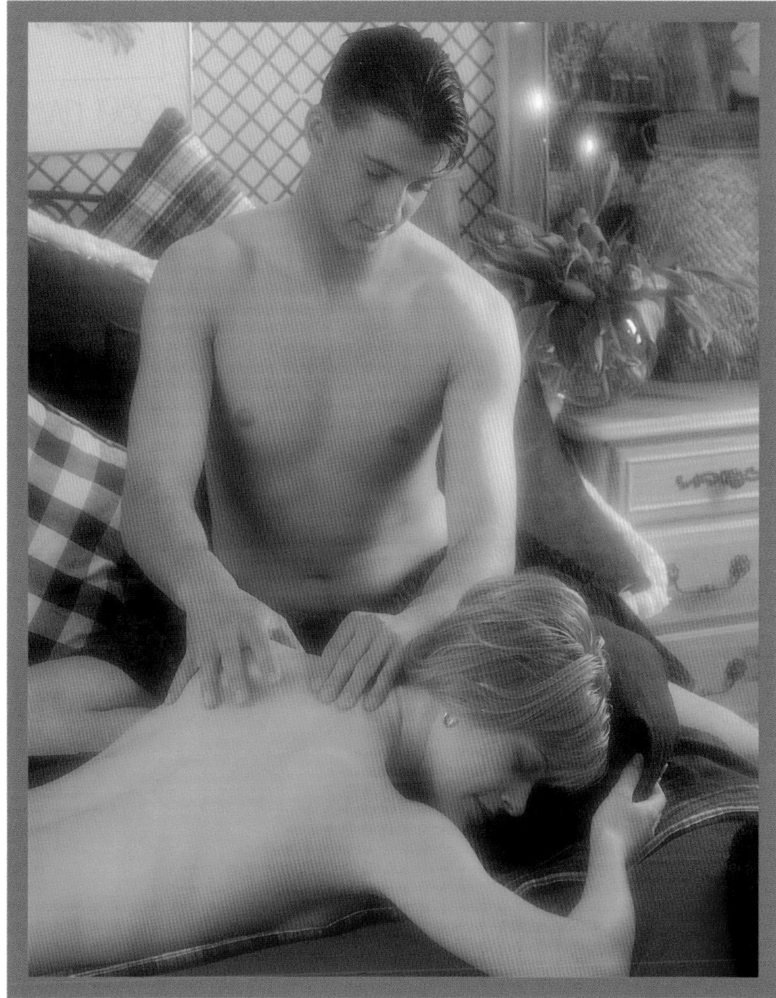

4 Continue the petrissage stroke all the way down the back, anywhere there is plenty of flesh and muscle. This stroke does not feel good over bony areas, so avoid the spine and shoulder blades. However, it is a wonderful sensation to knead the back muscles to just above the buttocks and back up again to the shoulders. As you finish your petrissage strokes, you may want to use nice deep effleurage to the back as an introduction to your next set of strokes to the back.

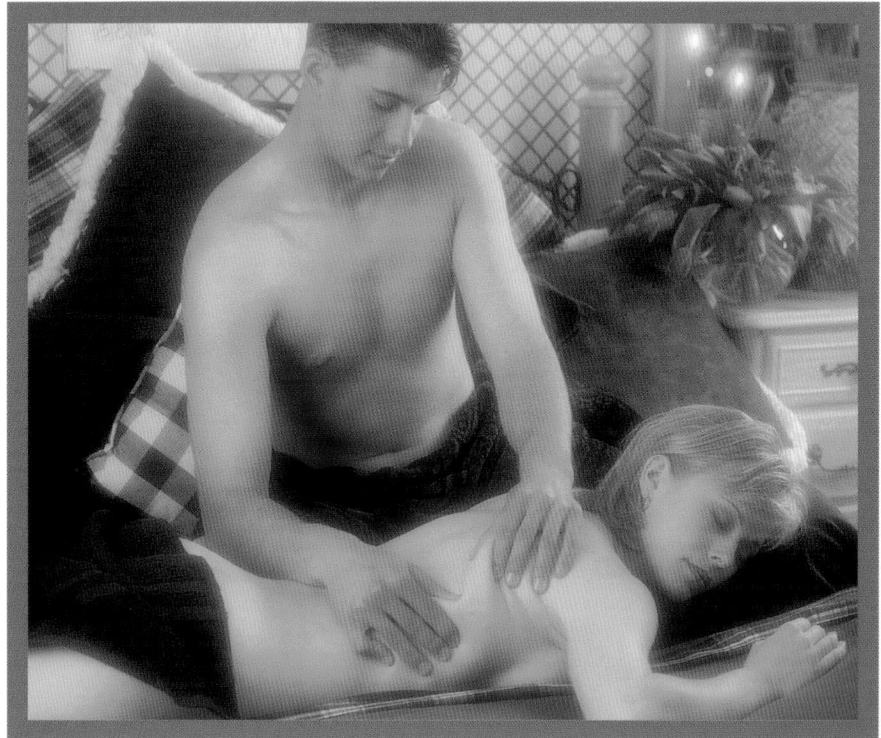

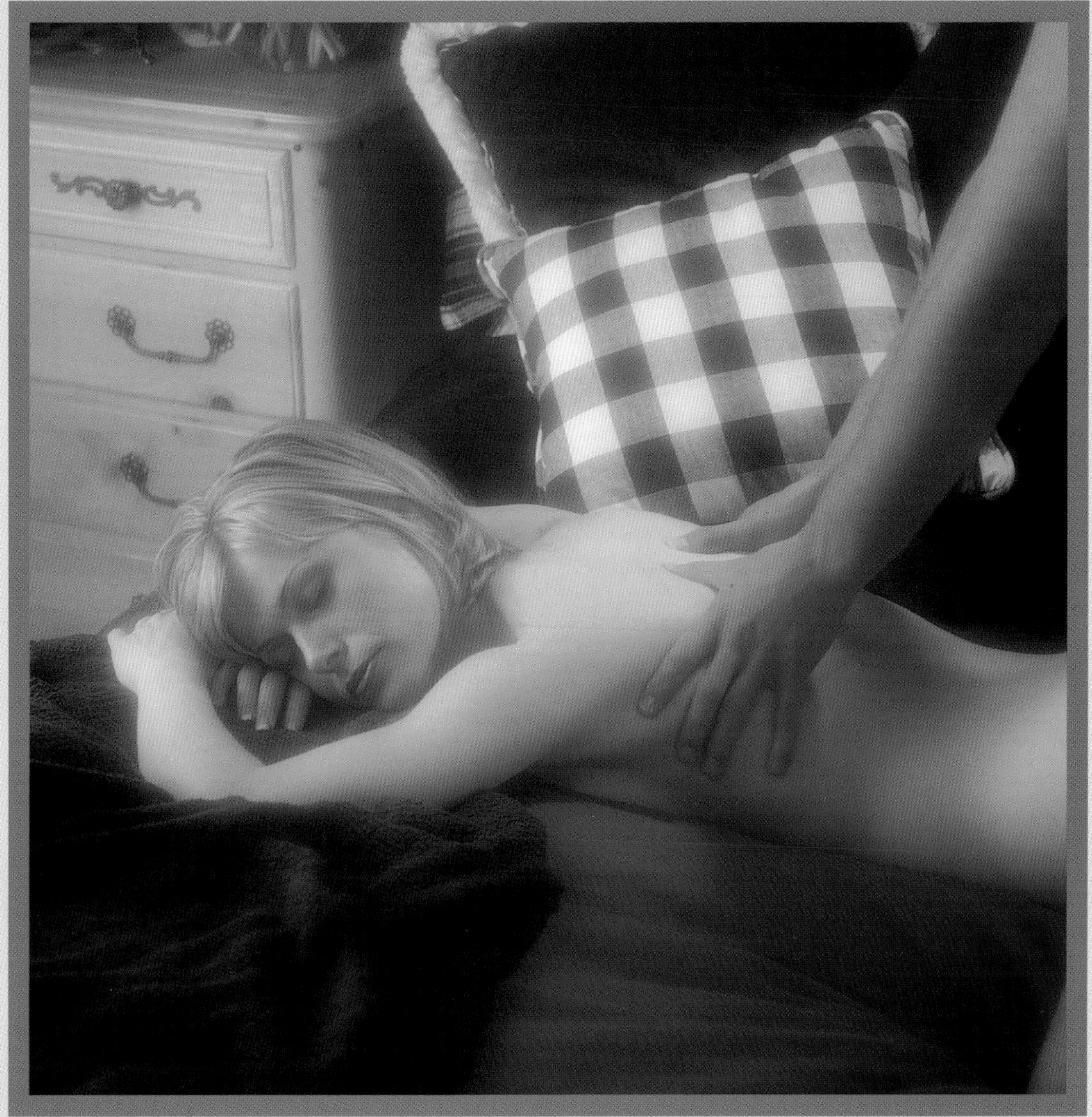

5 Position your hands between the shoulder blades. Use thumb compression or pressing approximately 1-2" from the spine on the large muscle ridge that supports the back. Press in gently and gradually with your weight as your partner exhales. Move down about 1" and repeat the sequence down the entire back, from between the shoulder blades down to and including the buttocks. Make additional passes down the back using increasing pressure and circular friction with your thumbs. These compression and circular friction strokes will smooth out and stretch away muscle stiffness, leaving your partner extremely satisfied.

5a This thumb pressure and circular friction routine is the basis behind Shiatsu, an acupressure massage from Japan. Japanese Shiatsu to the back requires no oils or lotions. It works on the premise that the body's life force, called chi, flows through invisible pathways or channels, called *meridians*, over the entire body. When chi flows uninterrupted through these channels, you experience health and vitality. However, when there is a blockage of chi, there is a deficiency on one side of the blockage and an excessive buildup of chi on the other. This blocked energy will manifest in the body as aches and pains, and eventually as disease. Massaging these ancient acupoints with thumb or finger pressure breaks the blockage and restores health.

6 Next, you can massage even deeper with an "ironing" stroke. Ironing is a blend of deep effleurage and friction because the stroke is long and flowing while deep and heat producing. Ironing is a very pleasurable stroke. You may use the flat of your hands or knuckles, or both, to go deeper. The stroke begins at the gluteal crack and proceeds slowly up the back on either side of the spine. Follow the contours and curves of your lover. Watch as muscles seem to melt before your stroke.

6a When using knuckles, be certain to use only partial knuckles as you pass between the shoulder blades. This is a narrowing between two bony areas and knuckling could hurt. Your return stroke should be light feathering to offset the deeper ironing. This produces a tingly sensation.

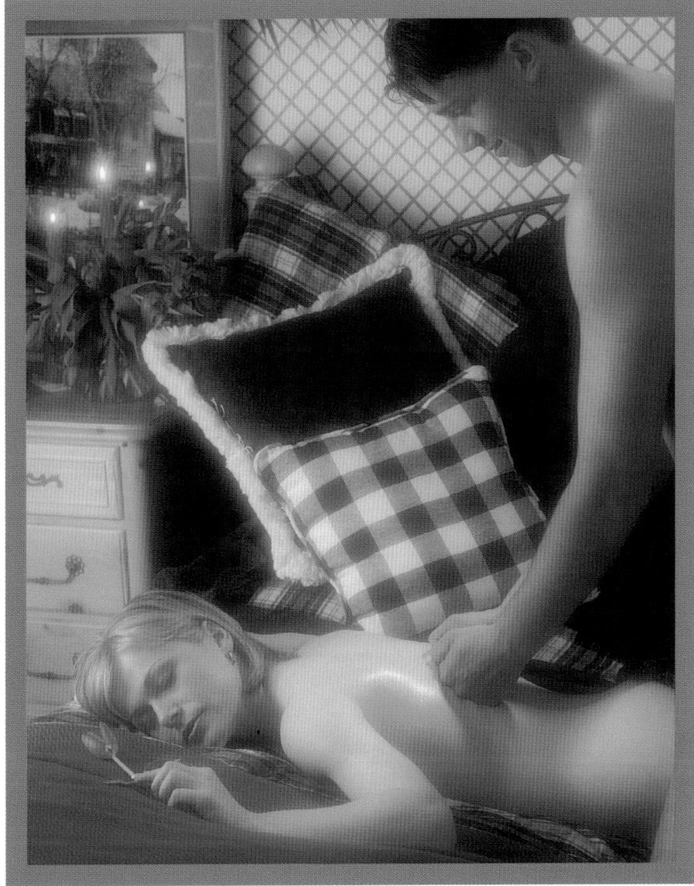

7 If, when you are using long deep strokes on the back, your partner mentions a particularly achy area, you could try a combination of friction strokes to this sore spot. Take a minute or two to apply pressure to find the exact location of the knot of tension. Use circular friction to determine the boundaries of the muscle tension; knowing how large an area you are working with can help you decide which strokes to use next. You could use a blend of kneading, more circular friction, vibrating, hacking, or plucking with two hands. Always end deep massage work with lighter strokes to relax the area before moving on.

99% of all women love flowers.
- ♥ *Buy her one rose.*
- ♥ *Bring her a bouquet.*
- ♥ *Select her favorite flower.*

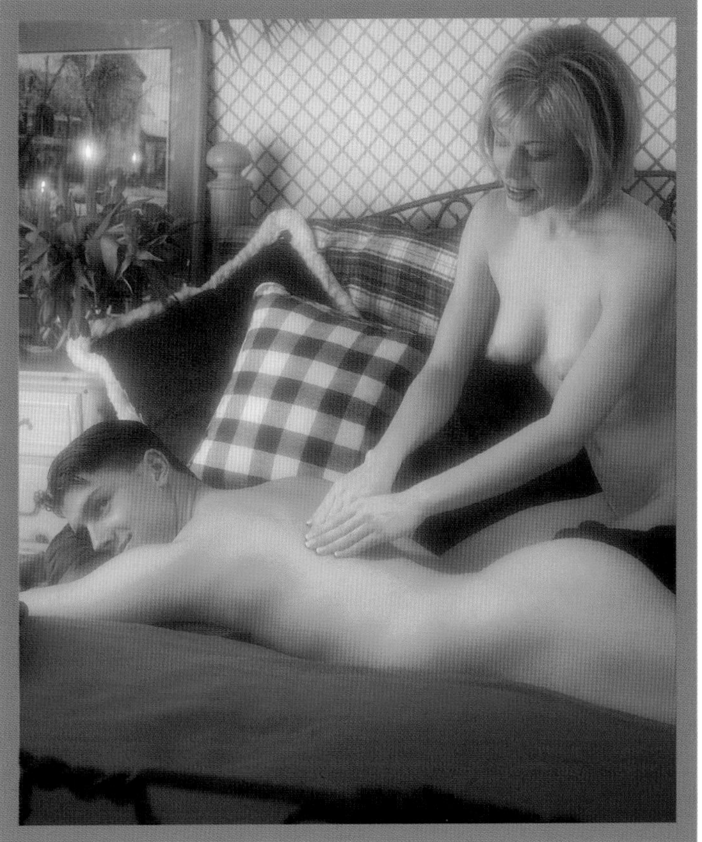

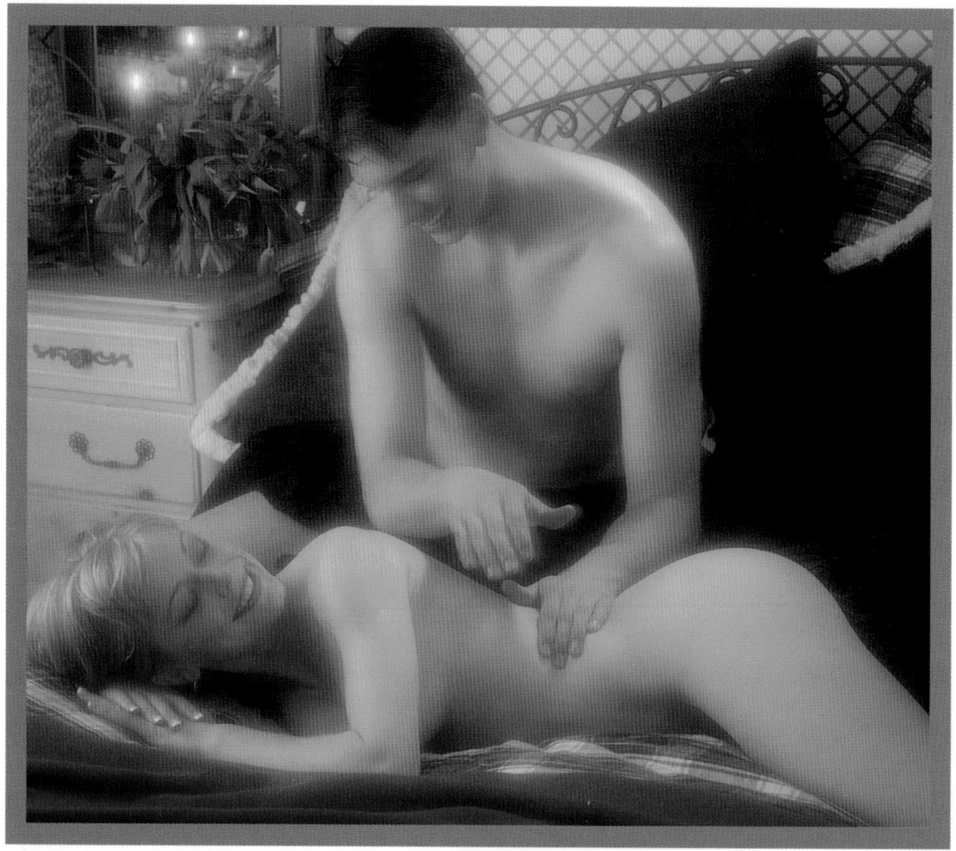

8 As you slip off to the side of your partner, you will begin to milk their sides. Reaching across to the far side of your partner, use long flowing strokes just above the hips and continue slowly up the ribs and down again. With each stroke, gently tuck your fingers against the flesh just under the bed line, then pull up and toward you until just past the spine. Place your other hand 1 - 2" above where the first stroke started and begin again. Repeat this several times on each side of your partner's body.

9 While at their side, use cupping techniques on the entire back. Begin adding light pressure to your cupping. Increase pressure over only the large fleshy areas, even though cupping is safe to use over bony or tender spots. This form of percussion helps to strengthen muscles while it nourishes and beautifies the skin. In addition to bringing blood to the skin's surface to give it a rosy glow, lymph fluid movement increases too. The lymph system produces and stores lymphocytes, white blood cells that help fight disease in the body.

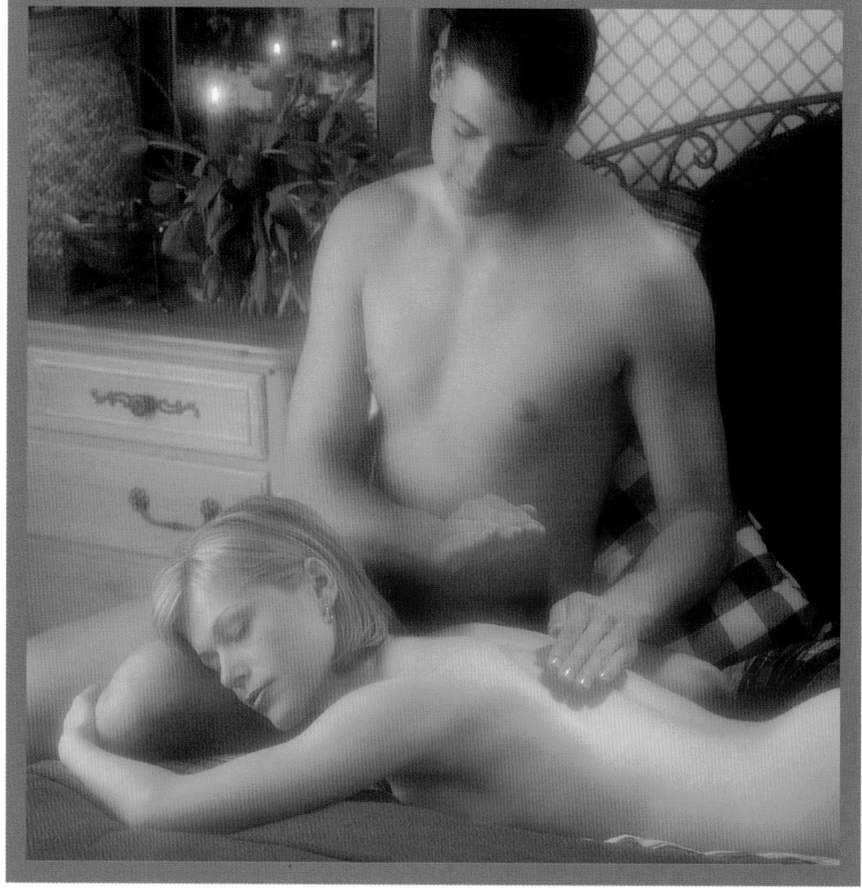

10 The last massage stroke for the back is a body stretch. The stretch technique can be done on the back and/or the side of the body. It is considered an effleurage stroke because it is long and flowing. Use your hands or forearms. Begin in the middle of the back and move in opposite directions toward the neck and buttocks, as indicated in the illustrations below. The bottom illustration shows the body stretch done on the side of the body.

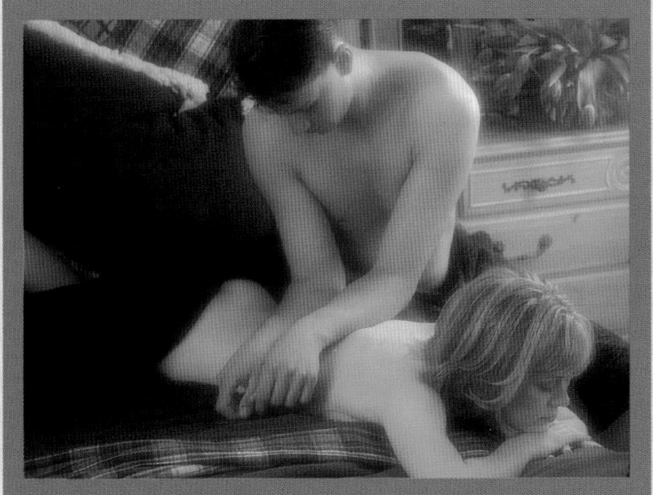

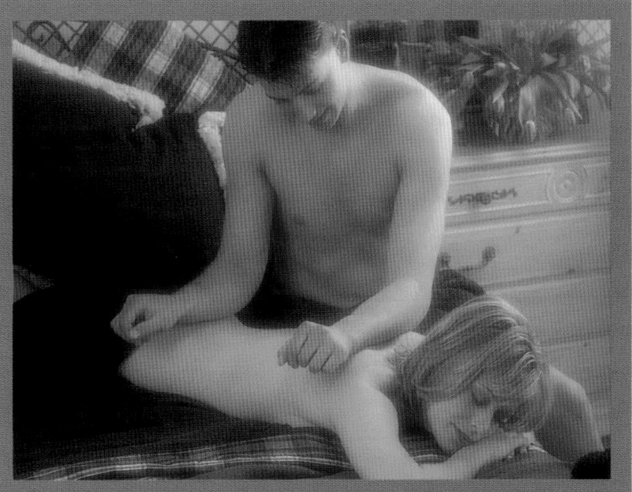

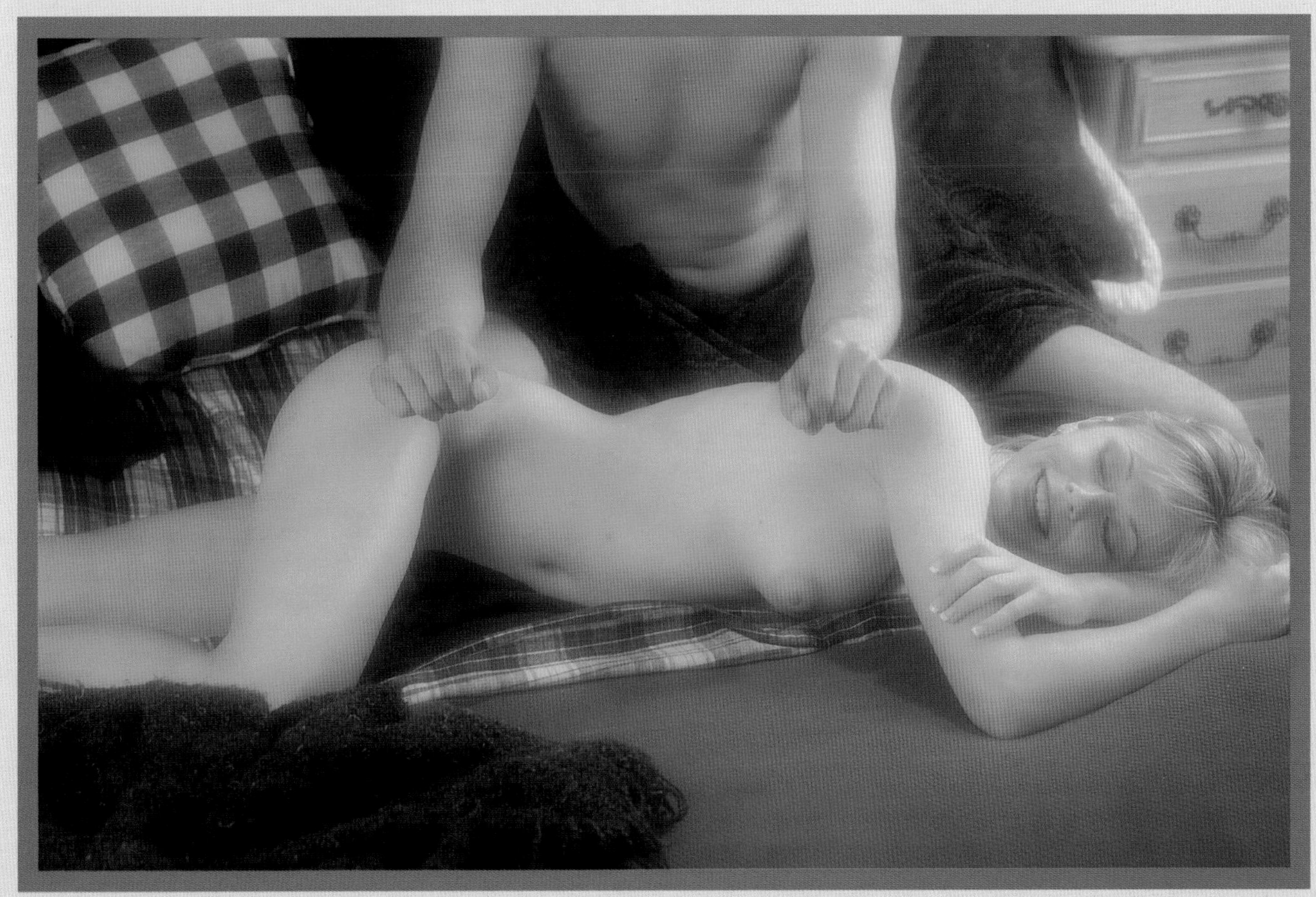

Massaging the Buttocks

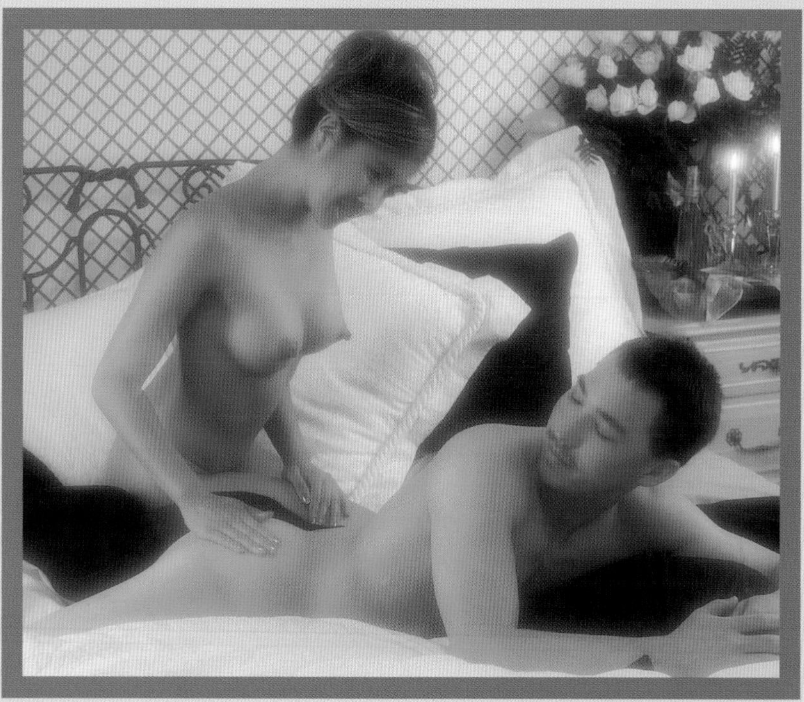

The buttocks are made up of several large muscles called the gluteals. They help move the legs for walking and climbing stairs.

1 Pour ½–1 teaspoon of warmed oil onto the back of your hand while it rests on your partner's buttocks. Take your other hand, scoop the oil, and begin with some long strokes down the glutes and up the sides of the hips. Then, sweep your hands in over the top of the hips, and repeat the stroke. Reverse the stroke, going up either side of the buttocks, up over the hips, and down the sides. Do this at least six times. Lean into the strokes to create additional pressure.

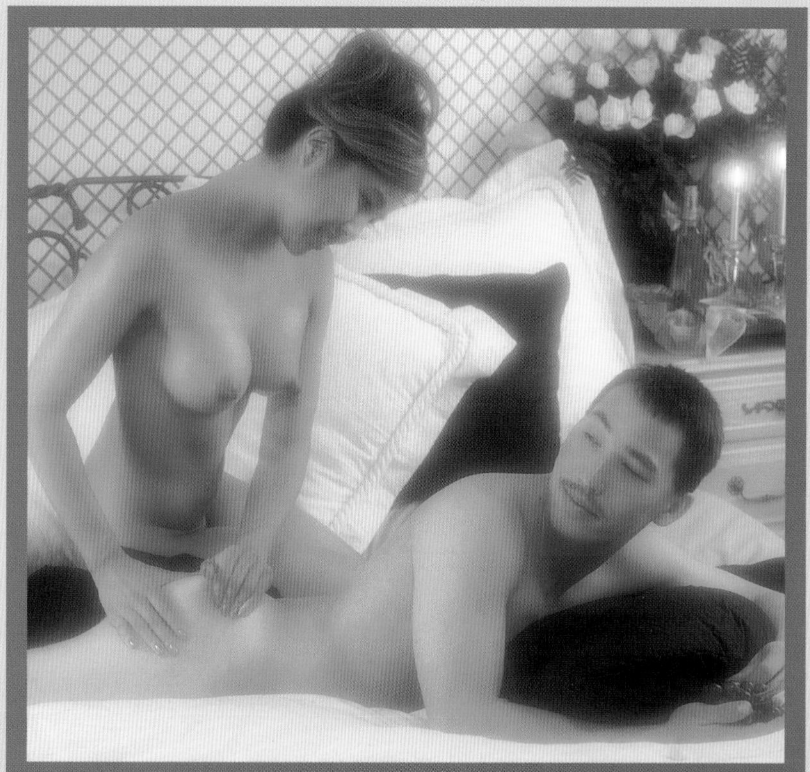

2 Now, petrissage your partner's buttocks. Grab the thick muscles between your thumb and fingers. Squeeze and pinch like kneading bread dough. Use both hands on one side and then the other. The gluteals are large muscles, so you can be quite aggressive in your movements. Unless your partner suffers from sciatica or hip pain, there should be no discomfort in this stroke.

2a A natural progression from kneading, because you are already grasping flesh with thumb and fingers, is the percussive stroke of plucking. As you grasp the loose flesh of the buttocks, pull up a little with one hand and then the other. Do this slowly and deliberately at first, then more quickly as you pick up speed. Pluck one side of the buttocks and then the other.

3 Position your thumbs near the tail bone on each side of the gluteal crack. Use firm thumb pressure, move up an inch or so and repeat the thumb pressure. Follow the outline of the hip bone, making presses in the flesh beneath this bone. There may be some tender points. Be gentle, but as long as it is not painful, continue with thumb pressure up and out along the hip to the side where the leg connects at the hip socket.

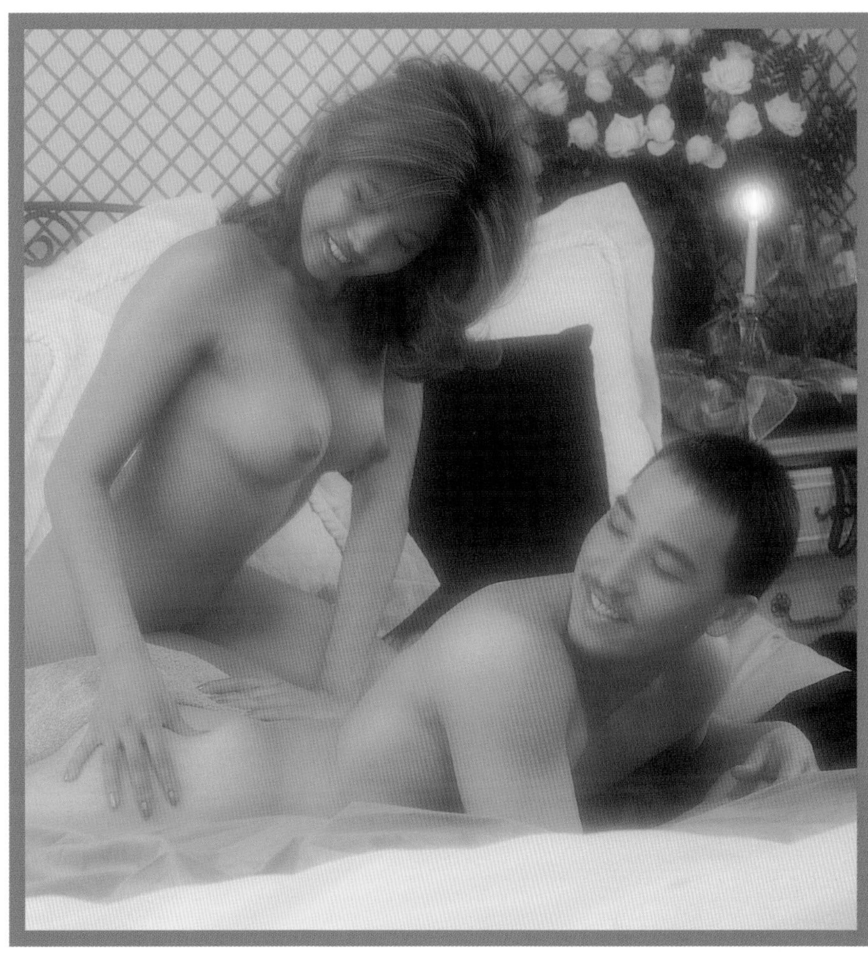

3a Make another pass or two using more pressure and circular friction with your thumbs or several fingertips together. You could even try using knuckles to press or make circles. This pressure is based on Japanese Shiatsu, breaking blockages to restore health. It is deeply satisfying for your partner to feel muscle tension released from buttocks, hips and pelvis.

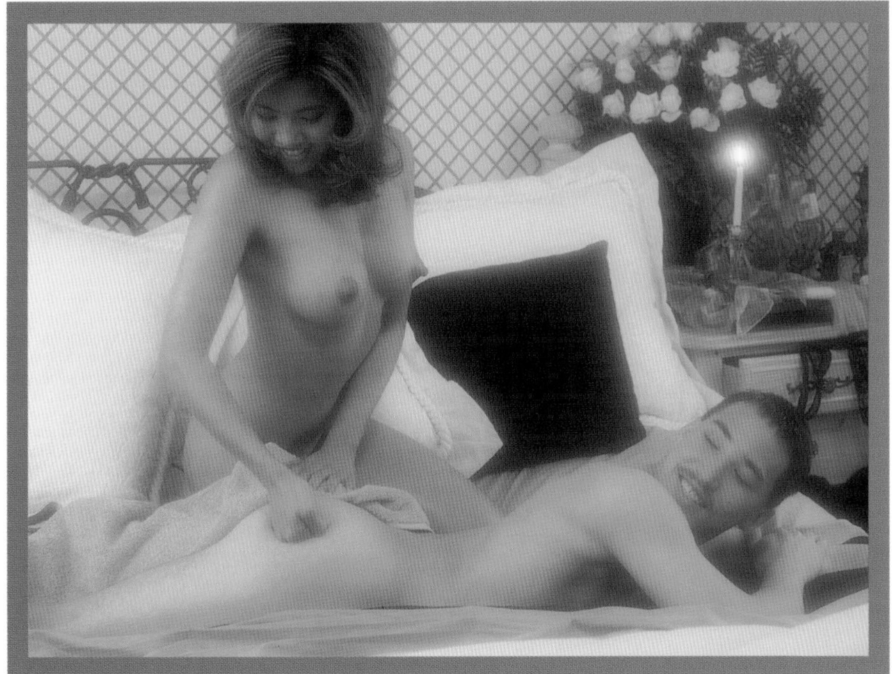

4 Next, you can massage even deeper with knuckles. Instead of following contours along the outline of the hip bone, begin massaging with knuckles over the entire buttocks. Be careful not to push deeply where you can feel bones; this will be uncomfortable. However, this massage stroke to the buttocks should feel great.

5 While at the side of your partner, you will use cupping and slapping techniques to the entire buttocks. You will want to begin by using light pressure, increasing pressure steadily. The slapping stroke you use will bring blood to your partner's skin's surface nourishing and beautifying the skin. The slapping stroke you use will also give a rosy glow to the skin.

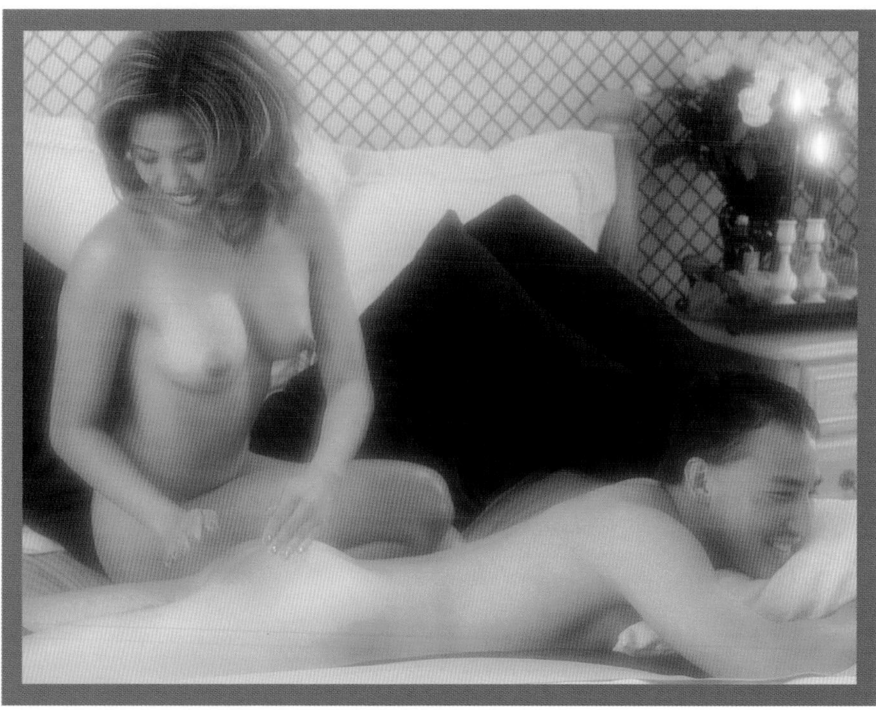

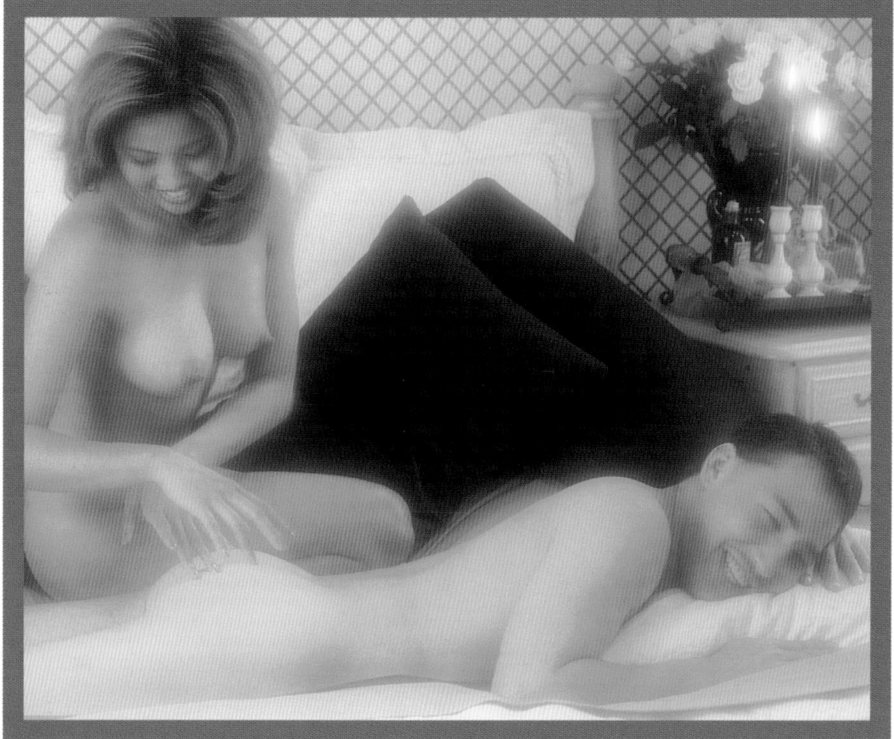

6 The last massage stroke for the buttocks is feathering. After the cupping and slaps, the ultra-light sensation of feathering will send waves of sensuous pleasure rippling through the pelvic girdle and then up the spine. The tingles may reach all over the entire body. Many people do not realize that the derrière is a major source of sensuality and eroticism. Take the back of your fingers (the nails) and lightly drag them up the center of the buttocks, brushing the gluteal crack. Move up and over the sacrum, and up and over the top of the hips. Then, sweep down the outside of the hips slowly with to the bottom of the buttock. Repeat several times. Try moving more slowly and lightly each time you feather the buttocks with your fingers.

When was the last time you were the seducer? How do you create the romantic mood? Are you playing the music, dressing the part, saying the right words, adding the little touches?

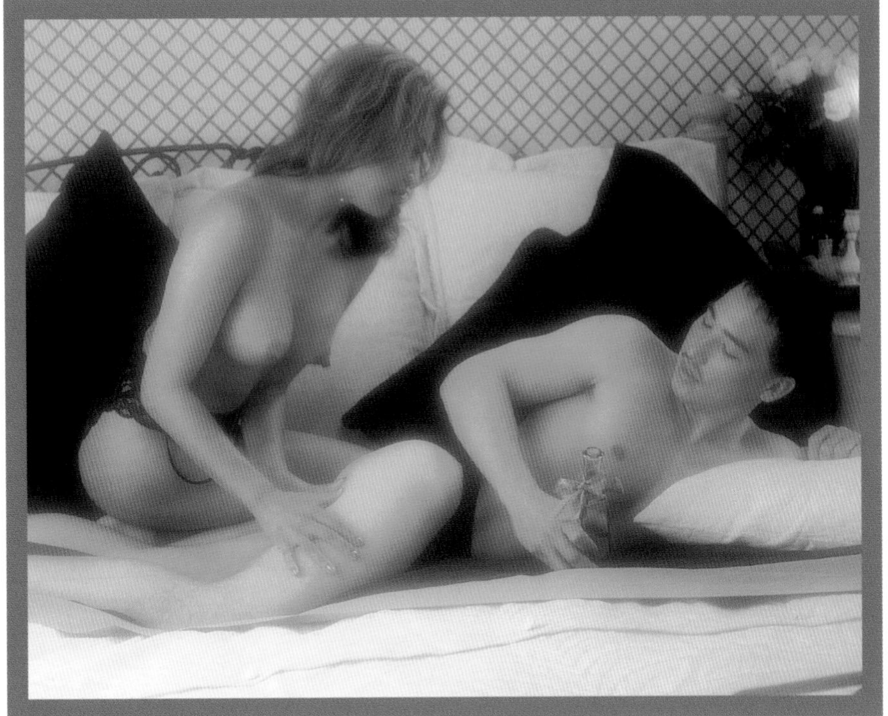

Leg & Thigh Movements

Legs and thighs are often neglected; however, due to their importance to the body and the possibilities offered by including them in your romantic massage, we will focus on the calf muscle, achilles tendon, and the hamstring muscles of the posterior thigh.

1 Use at least 1–2 teaspoons of oil on the back of the legs. Use more oil if legs are hairy. Rest one hand on the achilles tendon and pour oil onto the back of your hand. Take the other hand, scoop the oil, and begin with long strokes up the leg and thigh. Avoid too much pressure behind the knee. Then, sweep your hands in both directions — out and over the side of the thigh and to the soft inner thigh — and return lightly.

Essential oils , carrier oils, and pre-mixed massage oils may be purchased in bath and beauty stores, health care stores, spas, or other specialty shops.

1a Continue to effleurage the leg and thigh. The thigh can take firm to deep pressure because the hamstrings get very tight and need to be lengthened. Use deep effleurage to the hamstrings, but remember to use light pressure on the return stroke. Inner thighs are among the most sensitive of the erogenous zones. You may want to capitalize on the moment to deliberately tease and arouse as you draw your hands down the inner thigh. Brush up against the genitals with your fingertips in an ultra-light, almost accidental movement. If you choose to repeat this tingly brushing stroke of the inner thigh, realize that your lover is experiencing overwhelming feelings of arousal. This leg and thigh sequence can be repeated a half dozen times.

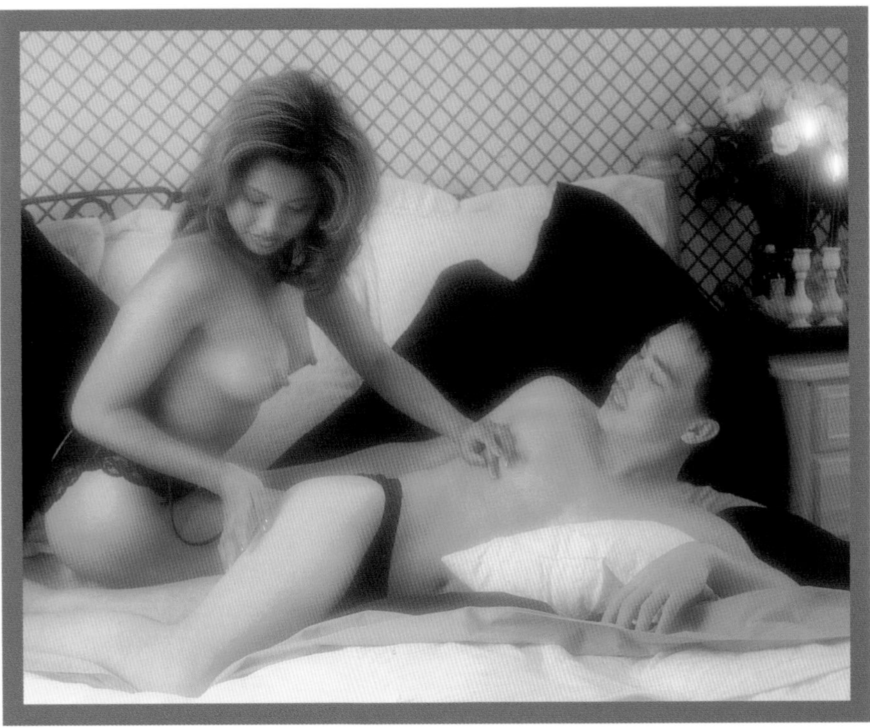

2 Petrissage your partner's calf muscles using medium pressure. Use both hands to grasp the thick muscles between your thumb and fingers. Squeeze and pinch in a kneading motion. Incorporate fulling strokes of the calf, before moving up to the thigh. Another stroke that you could use on the calf and thigh is plucking. As long as you are grasping flesh with thumb and fingers, pulling and lifting in a plucking fashion will help to loosen those tight muscles.

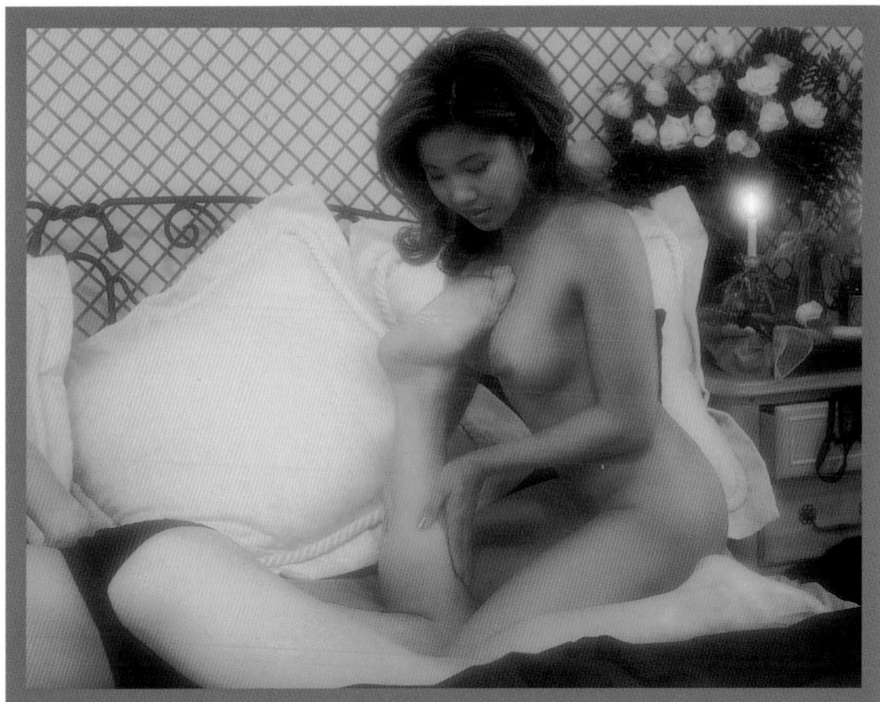

3 To go deeper into tight hamstring muscles, try using the knuckle ironing technique. Tuck your fingers under as if forming a fist, but leave the remainder of the hand open and relaxed with the wrist straight. Apply firm pressure to the thigh 3" above the back portion of the knee and continue to stroke up to and including the hips and buttock. Should you experience any discomfort or strain at your wrist joint, wrap one hand around the joint to stabilize it and add strength to the area as you stroke. This sequence can be repeated three or four times.

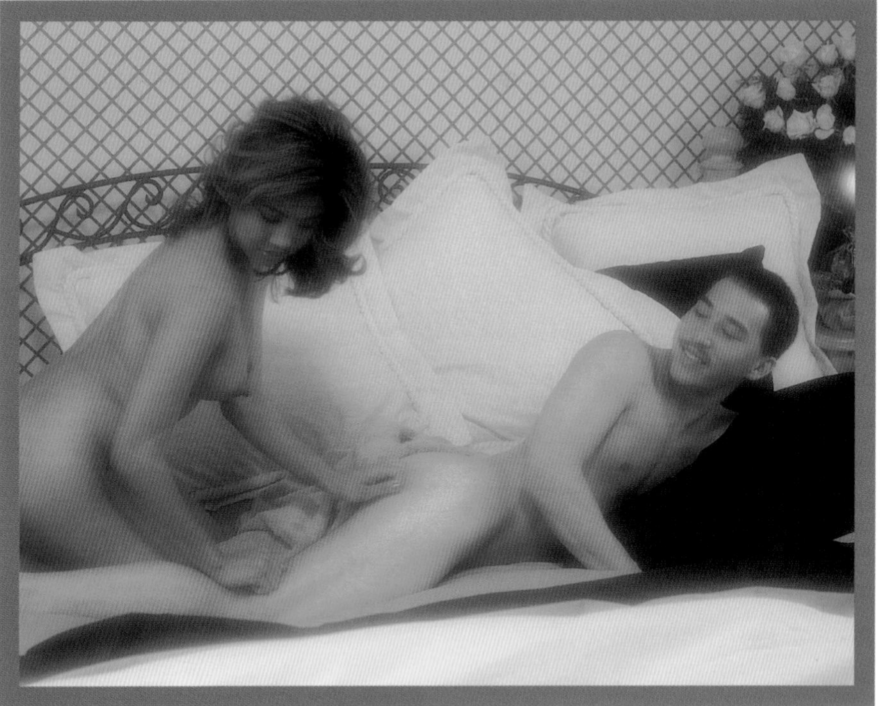

Refreshing Beauty Bath

1 cup chamomile ½ cup peppermint ½ cup rose petals 1 cup lemon verbena 1 cup lavender

The blending of these ingredients creates a relaxing, refreshing, and gently scented bath. Mix herbs together in a ceramic bowl. Place ½ cup of bath mixture into a 3" square muslin bag and tie with string or ribbon. Store remaining mixture in a sealed glass container. Run bath and add bag to water. Frequently squeeze bag to infuse essence into bath water.

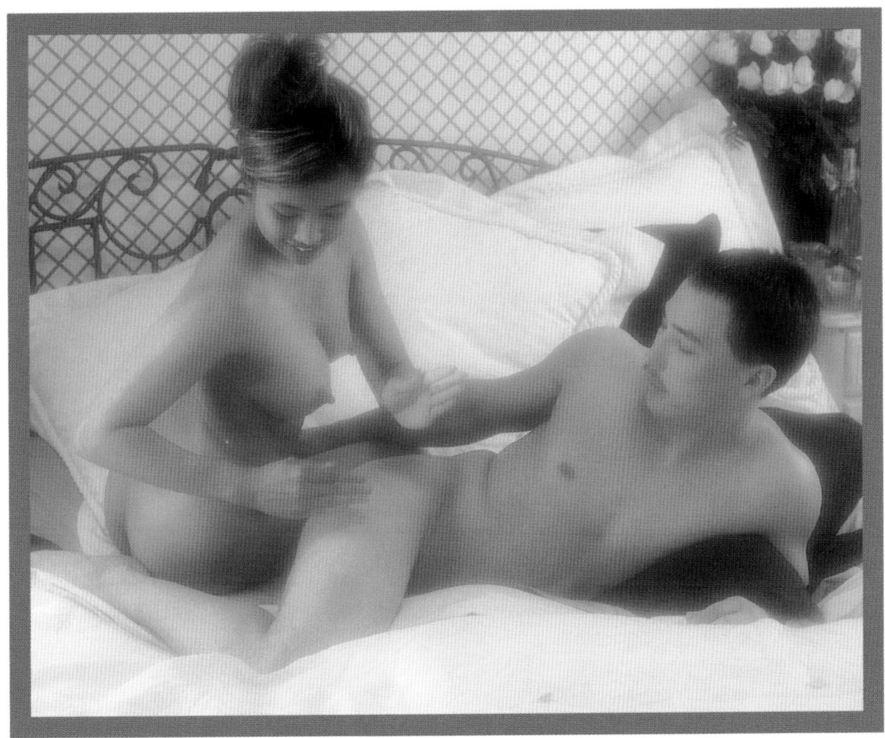

4 Percussive strokes are acceptable on the calf and thigh. Cupping, hacking, plucking, and whipping are all great to release muscle tension. Begin with light pressure, but increase steadily. The only problem with percussive strokes on the leg is that you may get tired arms while executing the strokes. That is why you should use more than just one type of percussion on the leg and thigh. As your arm tires from cupping, try hacking, then plucking, then whipping. Move back and forth, up and down the leg and thigh until the skin gets tingly all over and rosy in appearance.

5 As you finish both legs, feather both legs and thighs as the last stroke of the posterior limbs. After the more aggressive percussion strokes, a light sensation of feathering will tickle and pleasure your lover. Focus on the inner legs and thighs as you stroke up toward and include the buttocks. Drag the backs of your fingers slowly between the legs, and up and over the back portion of the knee. Focus on the inner thighs. Brush very lightly up against the genitals as you continue up the center of the buttocks, brushing the gluteal crack. Move up and over the sacrum, and up and over the top of the hips. Then, sweep down the outside of the hips slowly with your fingertips to the bottom of the legs. Repeat this several times. Slow down your last pass; linger in those sensitized areas.

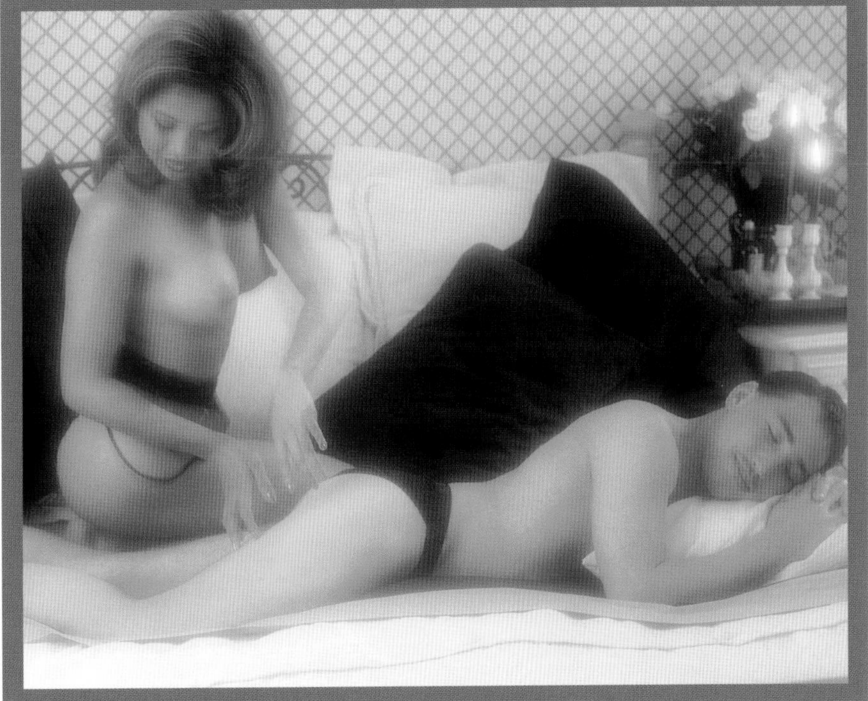

Do you know where your partner's "Love Buttons" are?
"Love Buttons" are those special things you do or say that bring happiness to your partner. They are the sensitive and sentimental opportunities you use to please that person special to you.

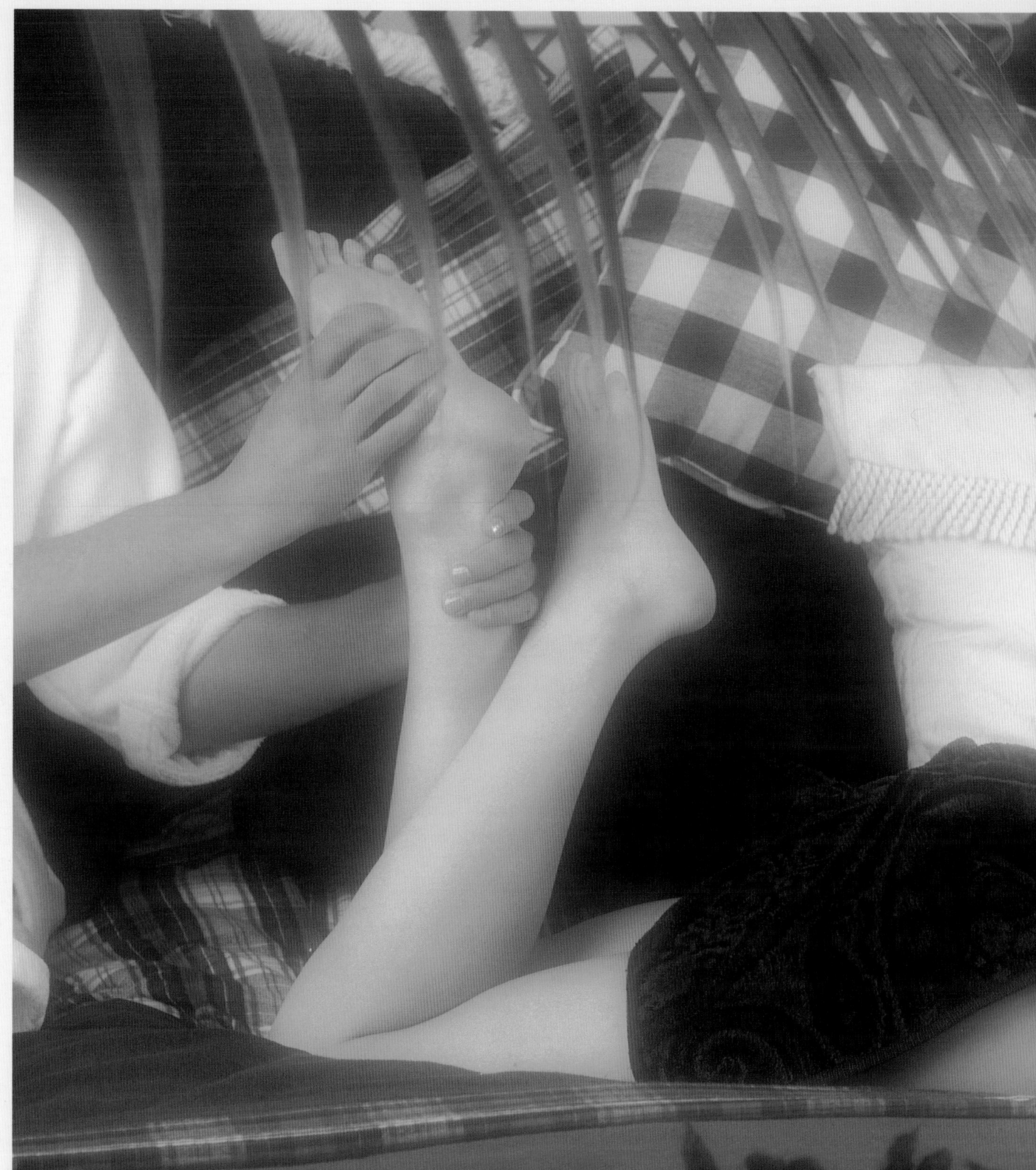

Touch. Explore. Enjoy the pleasure you both receive from each discovery as your hands linger with each massage stroke.

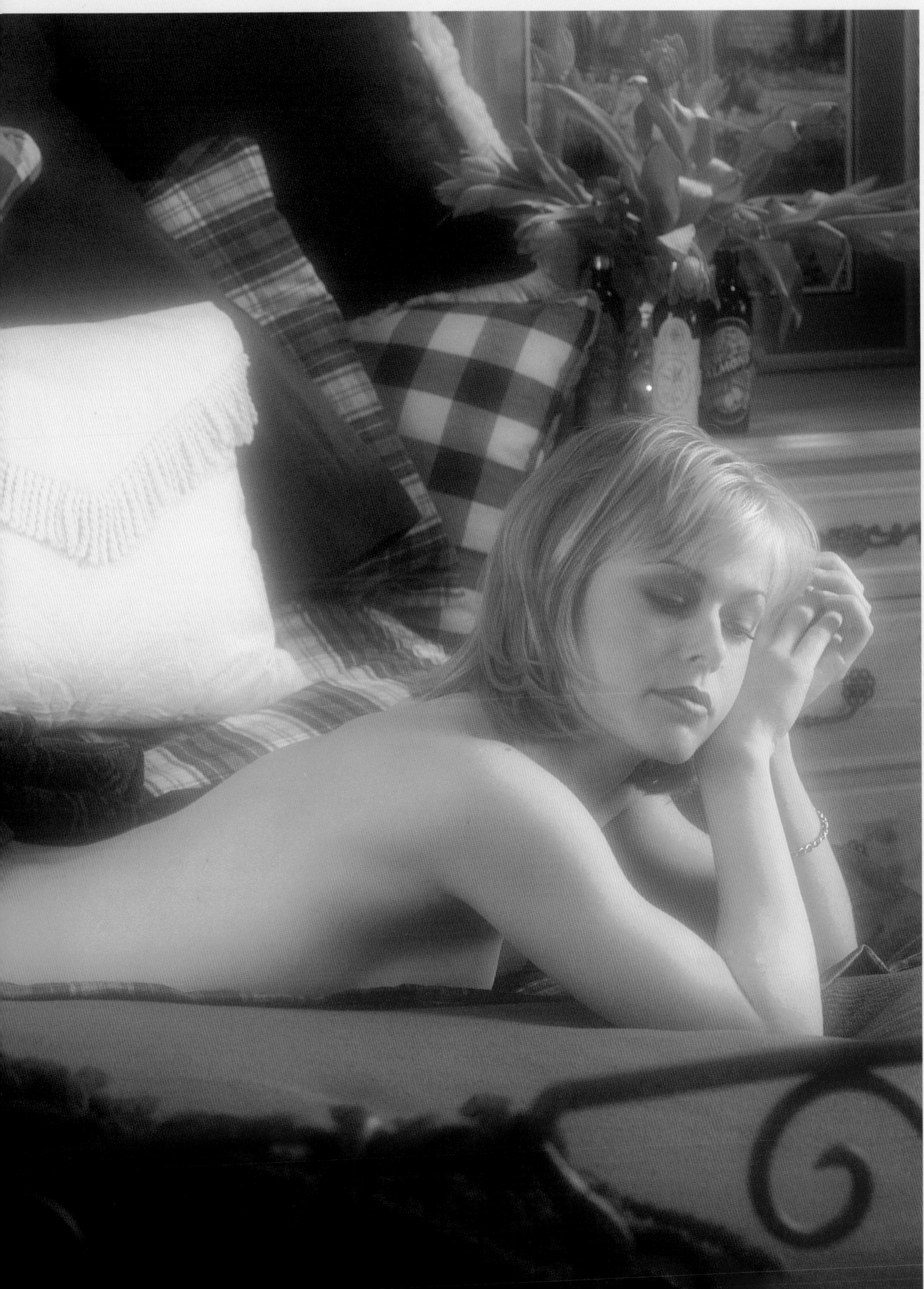

chapter six

Treat Their Feet

People, for the most part, abuse their feet, if not totally ignore them. However, feet carry the weight and, compared to the back and legs, have large numbers of nerve endings for the space they occupy. The more free nerve endings present, the more sensations and the more sensitivity. Yet, we allow toes to be pinched into tight shoes, feet to suffocate in confined sweaty places for most of the day, and stand or walk for long periods. All these will result in tired achy feet.

One of the best ways to get on your lover's good side is to treat them to a foot massage. The sequence for foot massage, as outlined in this chapter, is only one part of an entire massage. However, it can be modified to become a beautiful expression of love in and of itself. Review the section on feet and experiment with your special someone. If you perform this foot massage alone, as part of an overall massage, or in combination with a soothing foot bath after a long and difficult day, your lover will be a changed person.

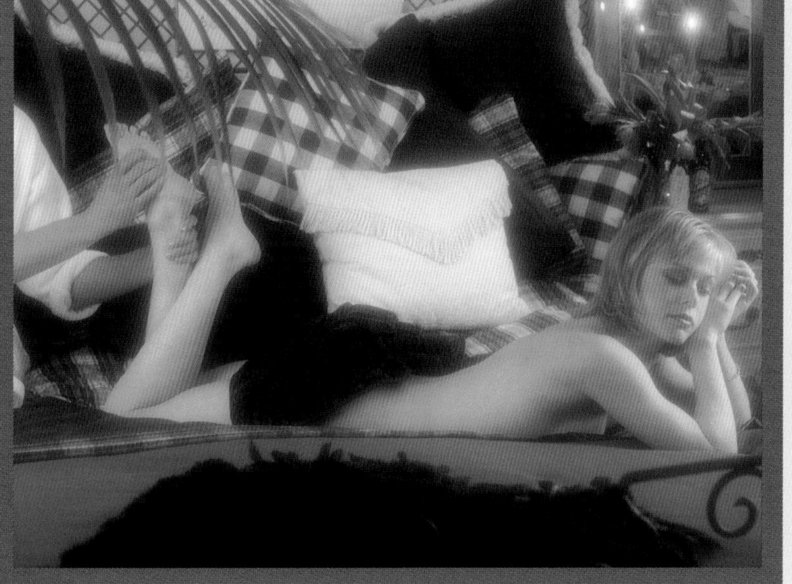

Feet are much more than just individual portions of the body that we often neglect. You can affect the entire body by just massaging the feet. The feet are the mirror of the body. So, if you have back problems, it will be reflected in the feet. If you have a digestive disorder, it too will be reflected in the feet. This concept of the whole body being reflected or mapped on the feet is called **reflexology.** It is a systemized massage, focusing on the feet, that promotes health.

Mix a foot bath for your lover. Fill a basin with warm water using a commercial scented bath salt or one of the following formulas:

Relaxing Foot Bath

4 drops myrrh oil   4 drops chamomile oil   4 drops orange oil   3 drops lemon oil   1 tsp. carrier oil

Rejuvenating Foot Bath

4 drops eucalyptus oil   4 drops pine oil   4 drops peppermint oil   3 drops geranium oil   1 tsp. carrier oil

Bottom of the Feet

1 As you complete massaging the back side of your partner's legs and thighs, position yourself facing their feet. Apply sufficient oil on both of your hands to lubricate one foot and ankle. Lift the leg at or above the ankle bone with the bottom of their foot facing toward you. Make contact with your free hand as you sense their skin temperature, and ticklishness or sensitivity. If you both want to enter into some playful touches and tickles, this playful teasing between partners can be endearing and quite pleasurable. However, tickling someone who does not want to be tickled can violate their boundaries of trust

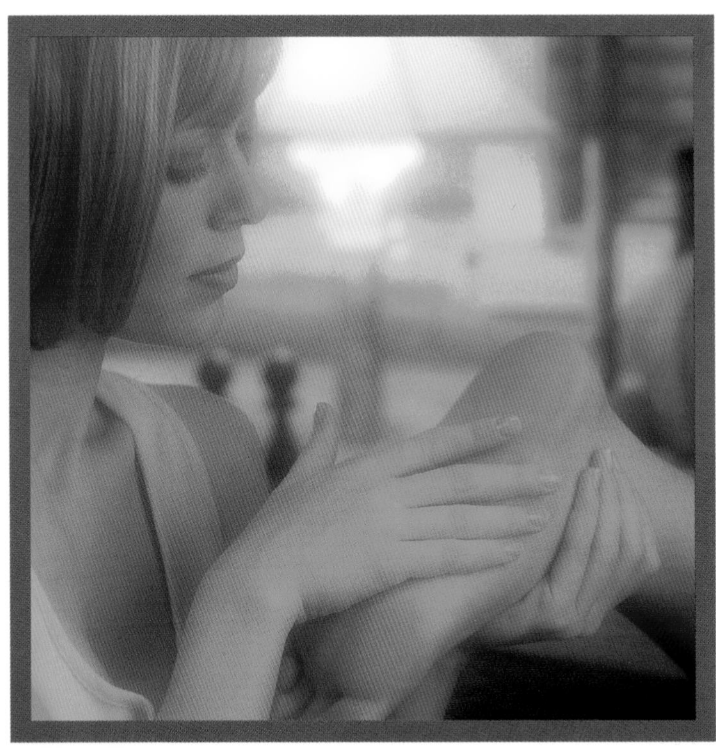

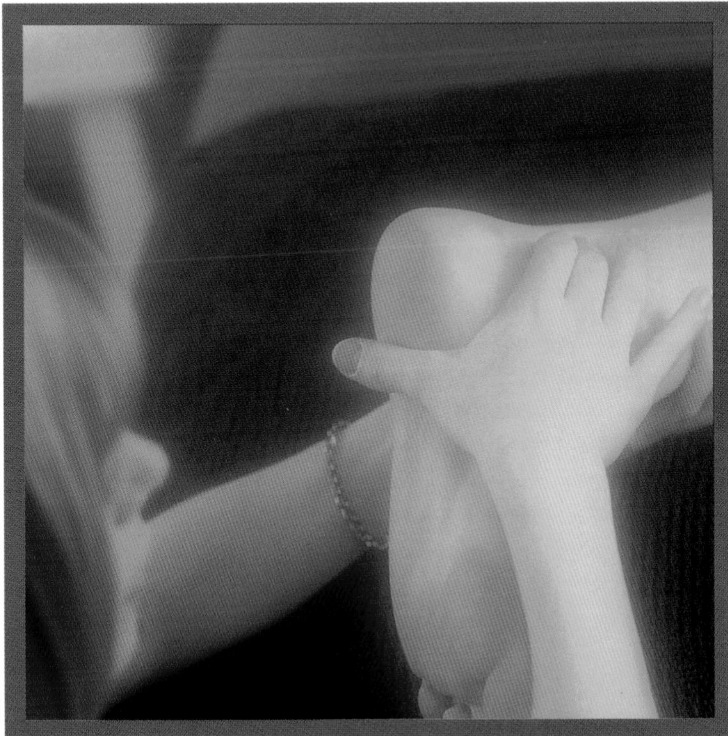

2 Using your fingers, run slowly and deeply along one side of the achilles tendon, just behind the ankle bone. This is one of the thickest and strongest tendons in the body. It extends from the base of the heel up approximately four to six inches, then disappears as it blends into the calf muscles. Tendons function like ropes that anchor down or connect muscles to bones both at the origin (where the muscle begins) and at the muscle's attachment (where the tendon crosses over a joint to make the skeleton move).

2a Switch hand positions and massage along the other side of this tendon. There can be considerable tension at the achilles tendon; massaging this area feels wonderful.

Romance on A Budget:

- ♥ *Flowers do not have to be expensive, try: super markets, street vendors, meadows, your own yard.*
- ♥ *Make your own coupon book: undivided attention, dinner for two, romantic massages.*
- ♥ *Create a custom card or a hand written note telling of your devotion.*

3 Take the palm of your free hand and place it squarely over the ankle bone. This feels very secure. Make circles with the palm of your hand over and around the ankle bone. Do this gently, do not make the foot wobble haphazardly. Switch hand positions, so you can make circles with your palm over and around the other ankle bone.

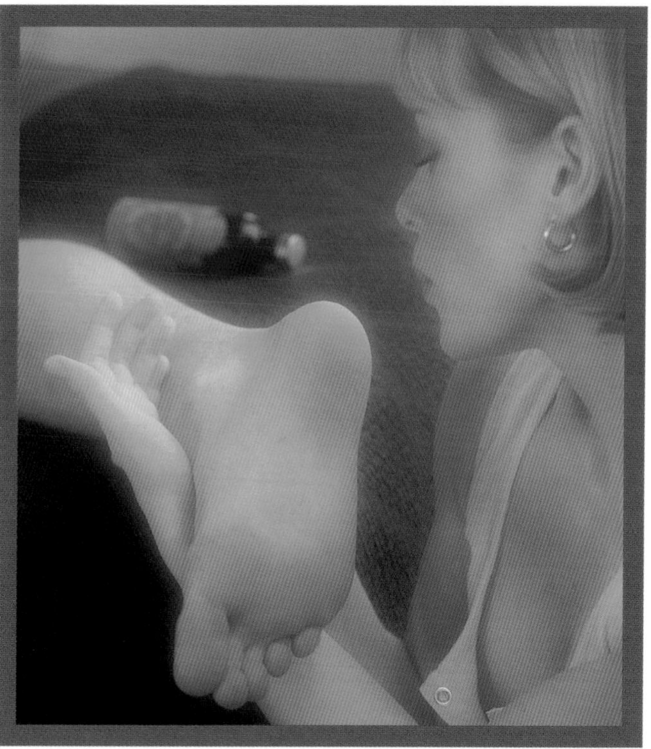

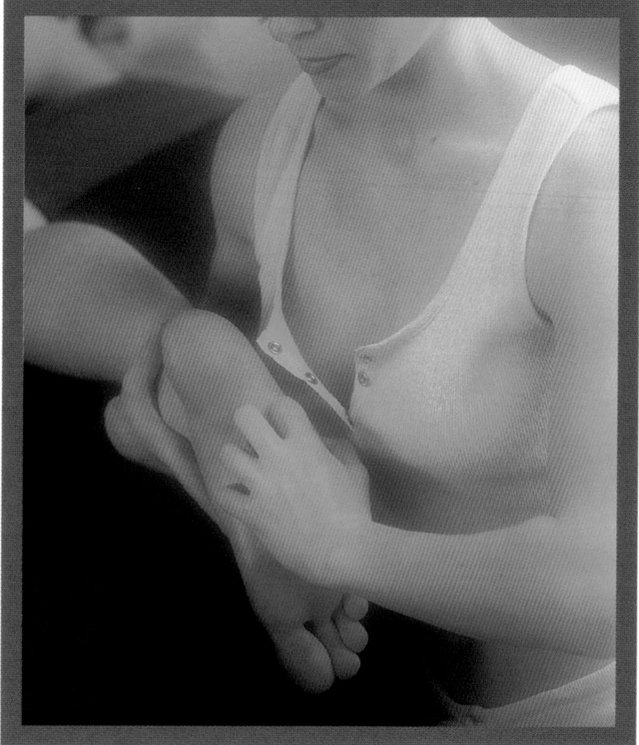

4 Make an open fist with your free hand. Knead the edges of the heel with the under portion of your knuckles. Knead the entire heel, both sides and the bottom of the heel too. Munch and crunch slowly and deliberately with your knuckles. This stroke and the next feel incredibly sensuous.

4a After kneading the heel with your knuckles, rotate your knuckles slowly down from the heel to the arch. Spend plenty of time here; most of the nerve endings are between the arch and ball of the foot. Gradually move on toward the ball of the foot and the fleshy part of the foot under the toes. Spend several minutes doing this.

Oriental Bath Ceremony

2 tbsp. dried star anise *1 tbsp. fresh ginger pieces*
1½ tsp. dried lemongrass *12 drops pine balsam oil*
Jasmine scented soap

Using a non-aluminum pan, mix lemongrass, ginger, and star anise with eight cups of water. Bring mixture to a boil and simmer for five minutes. Allow ingredients to steep for an additional fifteen minutes.

To set the Oriental Bath mood, change into a kimono or robe and burn a stick of sandalwood incense. Begin to mediate before you run your bath. Imagine yourself sitting on top of a mountain at dawn or the ocean at dusk. As you meditate recite this Oriental Bath Ceremony Meditation: "My bath is a time of absolute quiet and meditation. An hour of stillness and calm in the storm of my day. I will linger in my bath so that when I am ready to leave it, my mood has been altered, my inner balance restored." Once you are fully at peace, continue to meditate for five minutes..

Strain the herbs from the steeped water and, pour bath tea into your running bath. Add pine balsam oil to the bath and gently mix into bath water just before turning off tap.

Step into your bath and feel the peaceful energy that will refresh your spirit as you soak and lather with jasmine scented soap.

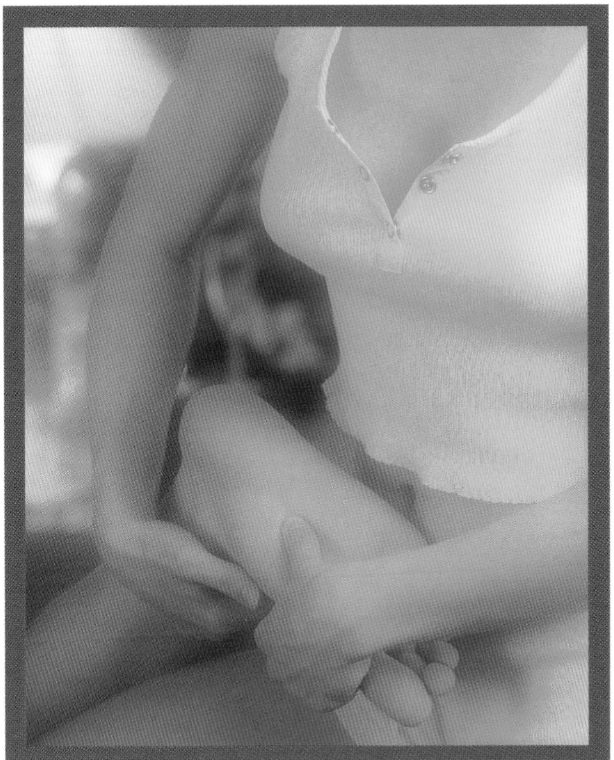

5 Now, use your thumb and opposing fingers to locate and glide down between the tendons, which control the movement of each of the toes. (You may exert firm pressure here because the skin is thicker on the bottom of the foot than anywhere else on the body.) Start just beneath the heel. Exert thumb pressure and glide slowly down the length of the foot to the space between the big and second toes. Repeat twice and move to the next tendon space.

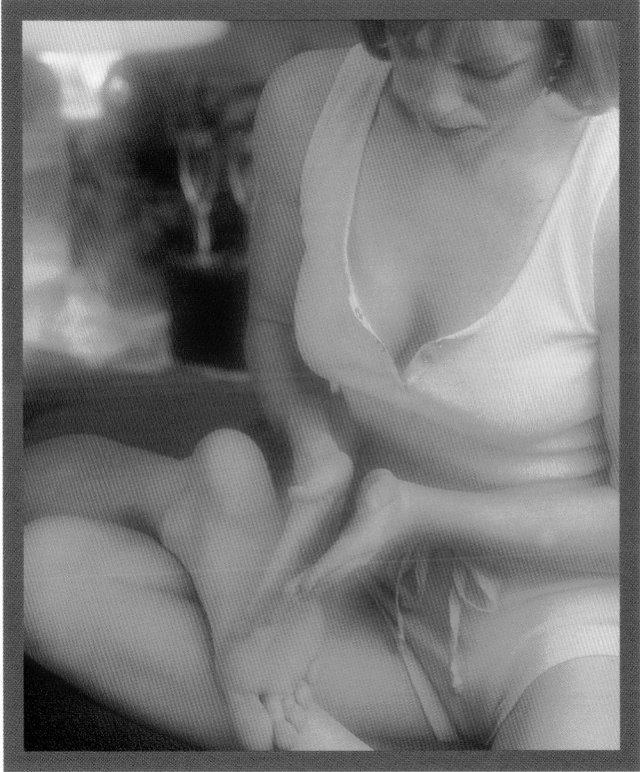

6 The next stroke to the bottom of the foot is a stimulating percussive technique that arouses the senses. Hacking the bottom of the foot is done with relaxed open fingers. Begin the stroke lightly and slowly. Steadily build the speed and force of the stroke. Once the stroke is fast and forceful, taper off the speed and force. Repeat this sequence of hacking to the foot until the bottom of the foot is tingling.

Some Oldie but Goldie Love Songs:

"And I Love Her", The Beatles
"Cherish", The Association
"Colour My World", Chicago
"Dream", The Everly Brothers
"Endless Love", Diana Ross and Lionel Richie
"Find One Hundred Ways", Stevie Wonder
"Hearing Your Voice", The Moody Blues
"Hello Again", Neil Diamond
"Just The Way You Are", Billy Joel
"Knights in White Satin", The Moody Blues
"Longer Than", Dan Fogelberg
"P.S. I Love You", The Beatles
"She's Always A Woman", Billy Joel
"Three Times A Lady", The Commodores
"Time In a Bottle", Jim Croce
"Unchained Melody", The Righteous Brothers
"Without You", Harry Nilsson
"You Are the Sunshine of My Life", Stevie Wonder

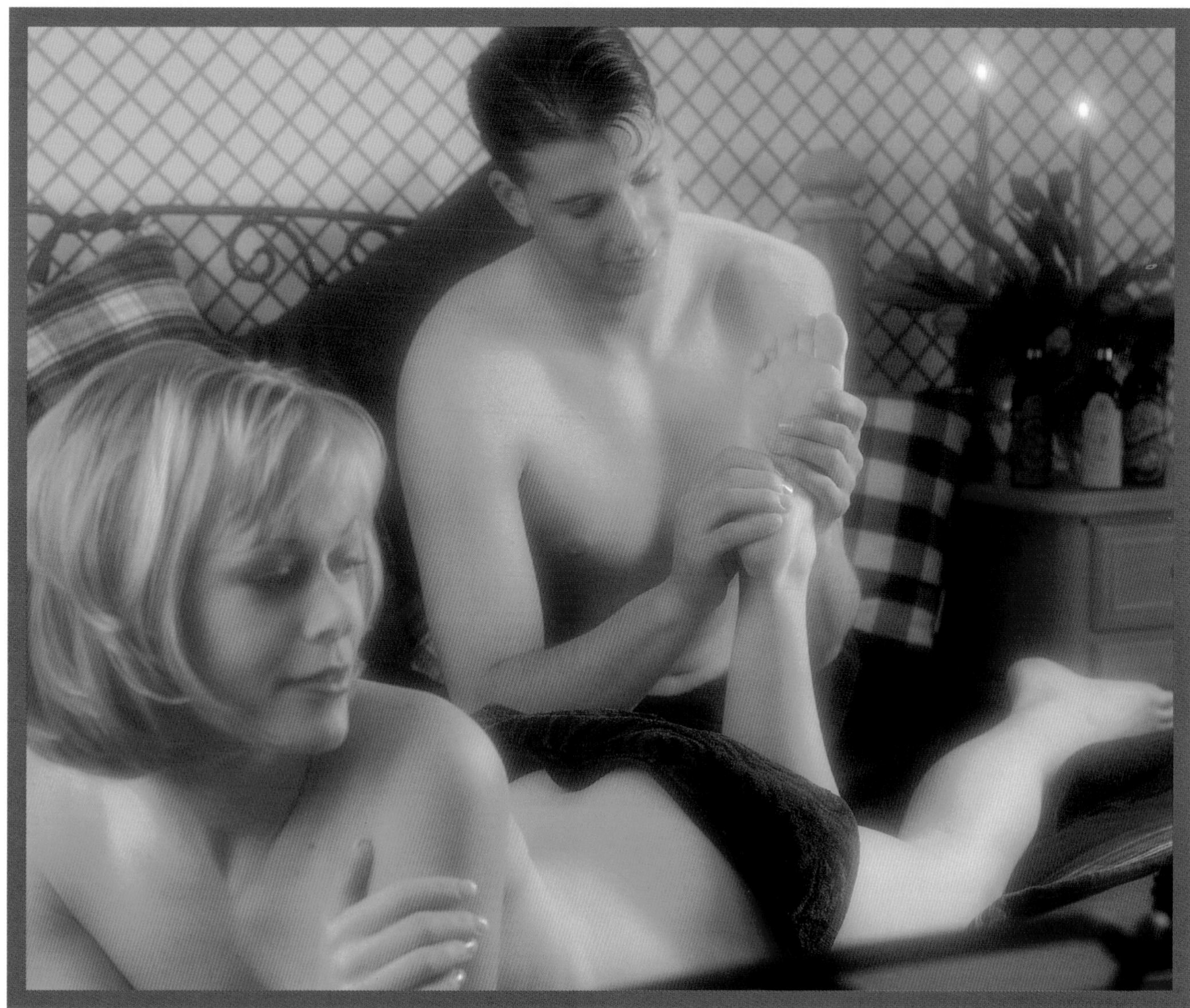

7 Finally, after your foot hacking stroke, it is wonderfully relaxing to soothe and pleasure your lover's foot with a series of long flowing effleurage strokes to the bottom of the foot. These strokes should be long and deliberate. As you slowly draw your hands, hand over hand in an alternating fashion, sense the tension being smoothed out. Feel your fingers slide off the heel, down the arch ever so lightly, and nuzzle between the toes. As each toe gently separates, allow your fingers to break contact, but only as your other hand begins to stroke the heel. Repeat this stroke until you almost lose count of the strokes because of the unending repetitions. You are now finished massaging the bottom of the foot. Begin the massage sequence with the other foot.

Having a hard time time thinking of a new romantic idea?

- ♥ *Brainstorm romantic ideas with your lover.*
- ♥ *Be innovative when making romantic plans.*
- ♥ *Come up with one new romantic idea each day and write it down.*
- ♥ *Set up a file to save your romantic ideas.*
- ♥ *Be on a constant look out for romantic ideas.*
- ♥ *Make a plan to initiate romantic ideas into a reality.*

Top of the Feet

When you are finished massaging the bottoms of both feet, your partner is ready to turn over for you to begin different strokes on the top of the feet. The skin on the tops of the feet is much thinner than the bottoms. You can easily feel the tendons for each toe. You may even see blood vessels. As you apply pressure, you may be able to feel bones beneath the surface of the skin.

With the bottoms of the feet, it is acceptable to lift the foot at the ankle. But, if you lift the foot at the heel while your partner is face up, undue stress is placed on the back of the knee joint; therefore, when massaging the tops of the feet, leave the heel touching the massage surface.

1 Apply a small amount of oil to the top of the foot as you make contact with it. Then, make long flowing effleurage strokes with your hands down the length of the foot. Separate your hands and allow them to circle the ankle bones on either side. Again, massage down the length of the foot and separate to wrap around the ankle bones. Continue this long effleurage, using your thumbs to slide between each of the tendons several times. Keep the pressure light to medium to avoid causing pain.

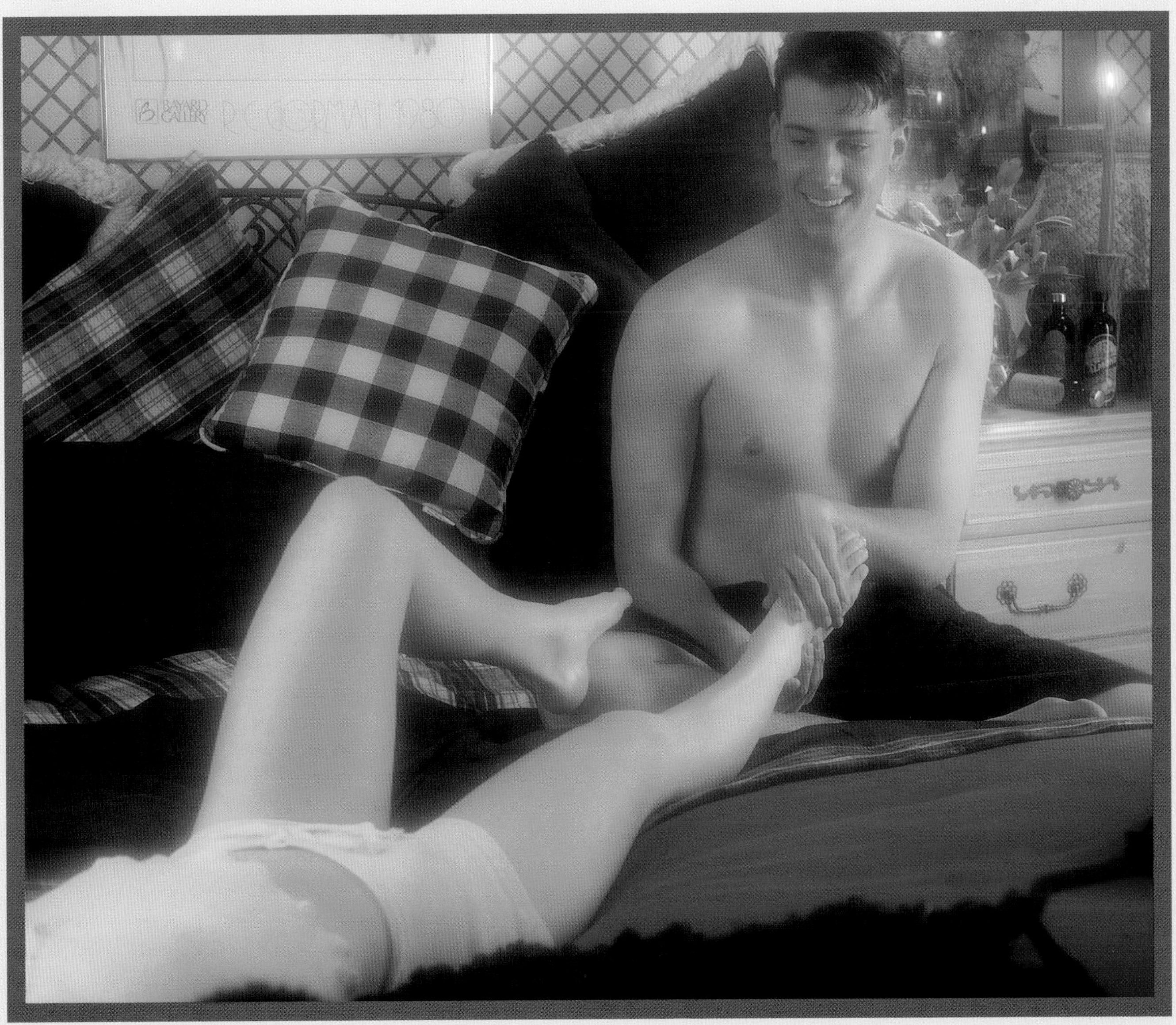

2 On your last time down between the tendons, create a bridge between this thumb stroke and the next one by effleuraging down the length of the foot again with a wrap around the ankles.

2a As your hands wrap around the ankle, fix your palms snug over and against the ankle bones. Move your hands back and forth in an alternating fashion, making certain to keep the palms from moving off the ankle. This stroke is a form of vibration called rocking. The main difference between rocking and vibrating is the speed of the back and forth movement. Depending on how rapidly you rock, the stroke might even be called vibration.

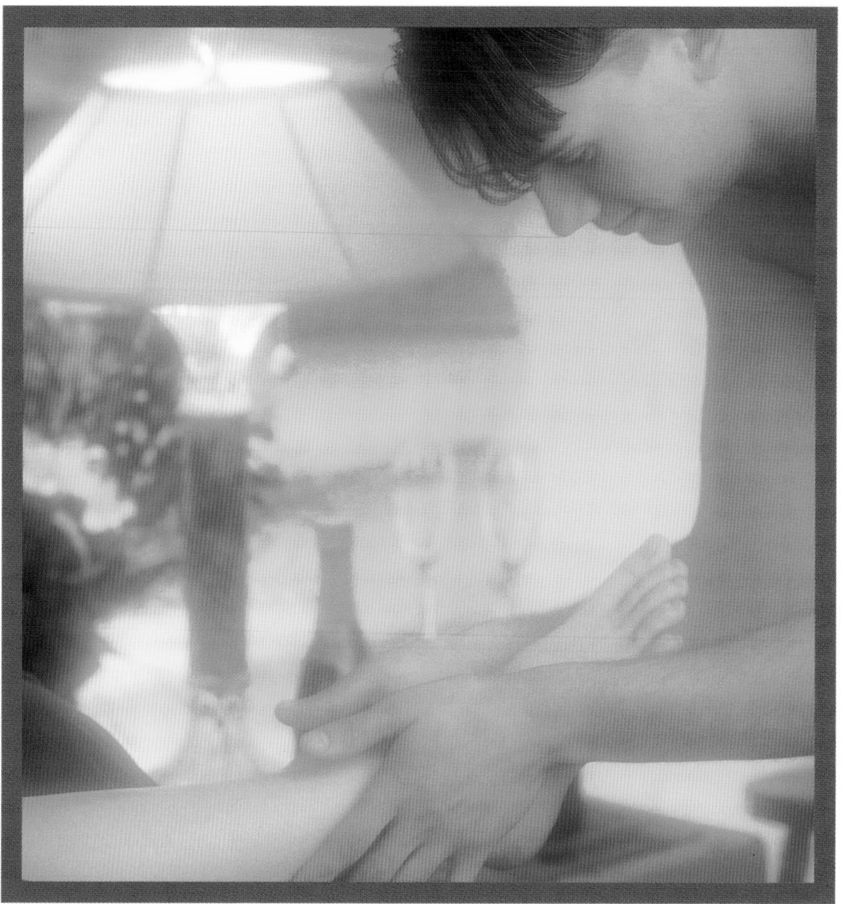

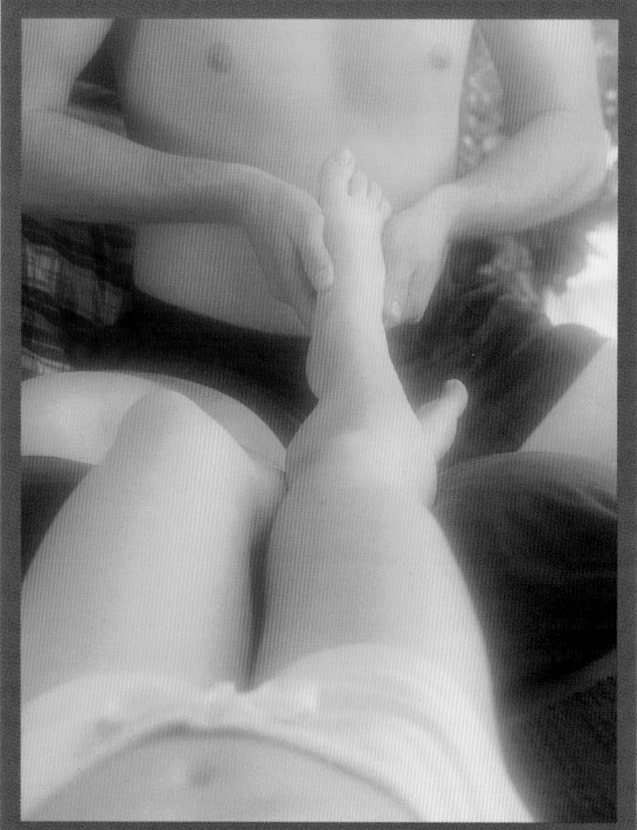

3 After rocking the ankle which creates a gentle shaking effect on the feet to help them relax, grab the foot with both hands. Place your thumbs across the top portion of the instep on the under side of the foot at the arch. Grasp the foot firmly, and squeeze. Push with the thumbs while pulling back with your fingers. This is called broad kneading or fulling. Repeat this technique several times from the ball of the foot down to the arch, but not including the heel.

Refreshing Herbal Foot Bath

Choose from: bay leaf, lavender, sage, sweet marjoram, or thyme. Place a handful of fresh or ¼ cup of dried herb with one tablespoon sea salt in a basin of hot water. When herb is infused into water, soak feet. To soothe itchy feet, add 4 tablespoons cider vinegar to your foot bath.

The Complete Book of Herbs & Spices

4 Move your hands to the arch side of the foot. Grasp the toes with one hand and place other hand above the ankle. Bend the toes down to flex the arch. The instep will be stretched at the same time that the arch is flexed. This gives your partner's foot an opportunity to stretch and flex, breathe and relax.

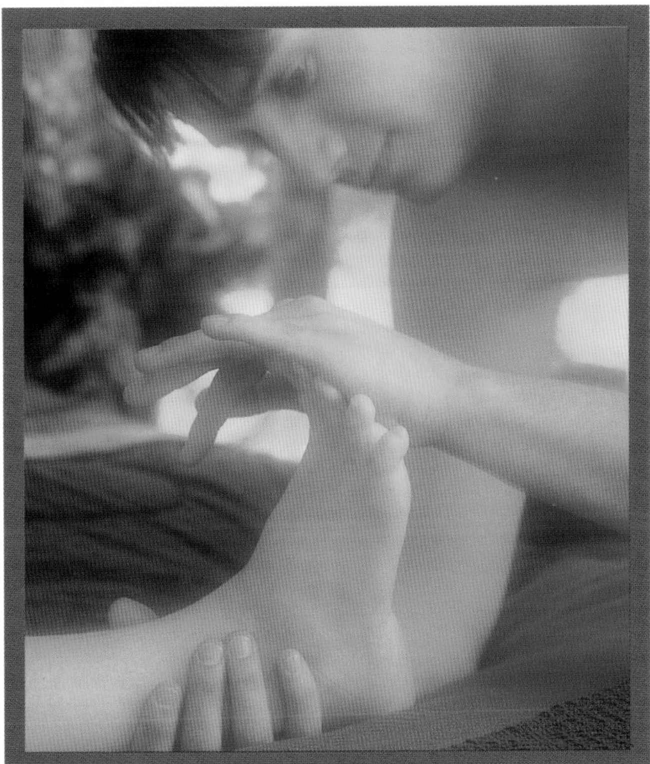

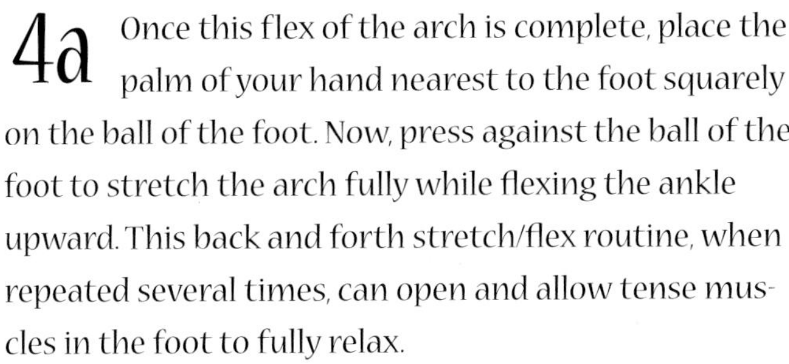

4a Once this flex of the arch is complete, place the palm of your hand nearest to the foot squarely on the ball of the foot. Now, press against the ball of the foot to stretch the arch fully while flexing the ankle upward. This back and forth stretch/flex routine, when repeated several times, can open and allow tense muscles in the foot to fully relax.

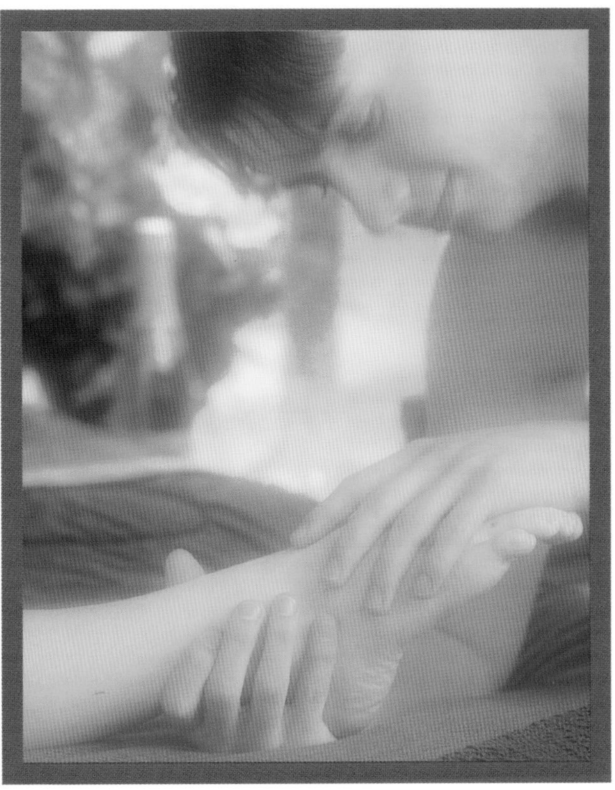

Glycerin and Rosewater Hand and Foot Cream

4 tablespoons glycerin *3 drops rose or geranium oil*
1 cup rosewater *4 tablespoons cornstarch*

Blend glycerin, rosewater, and cornstarch. Heat the mixture over a double boiler until it thickens.

Allow to cool, then add rose oil, stirring well. Pour into screw top jars and label. This can applied to hands and feet daily.

Tropical Paradise Bath

1-10 oz. can unsweetened coconut milk *10 drops gardenia oil* *10 drops amber oil*

Run your bath, add the coconut milk and swirl the water with your hand until blended into the water. Add gardenia and amber oil, swirling it into the bath. Climb in and experience paradise.

Before you run your bath, slice a fresh pineapple, sprinkle with coconut, and place it within reach of your bathtub.

Prepare a special tropical drink using champagne and heart-shaped passion fruit ice cubes. Scoop flesh and seeds from six passion fruit. Using back of spoon, press juice through a strainer into a bowl. Freeze liquid until solid. Pour champagne into glasses, add ice cubes, and enjoy.

5 Now, for some of the more sensuous sensations, we focus on the toes. As you continue to hold your partner's foot in one hand your thumb is on the arch, use your free hand to massage each of the toes slowly. Grab each toe between your thumb on one side, and your index and middle fingers on the other. Start at the base of the big toe and slide up the toe. Make a slow and deliberate cork screw motion all the way up to the tip of the toe. Repeat each toe three times, moving slower each time you repeat. Do this sequence on each of the toes. This part of the foot massage should bring delight to your partner.

6 Slide your little finger between each of the toes. Be certain you have sufficient oil to lubricate the skin, because too much friction will feel annoying and could destroy the sensations and emotions you are trying to stir within your partner. First slide your finger between the big and second toes very lightly. Make that slow and intentional cork screw motion with your finger all the way down until you touch the webbing. Repeat this twice, then move on to between the second and third toe, and so on.

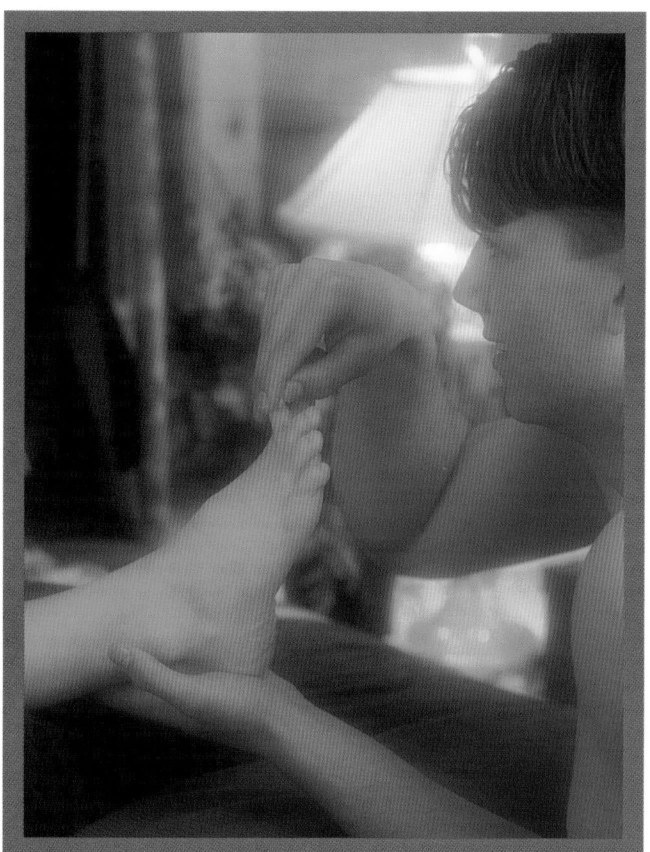

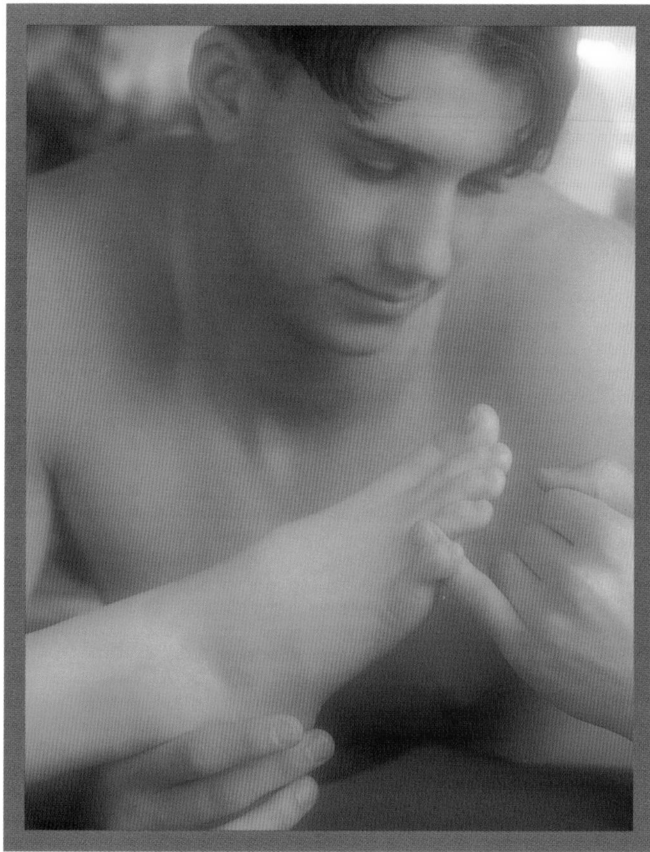

There are two kinds of romance:

- ♥ *Obligatory romance includes celebrating and purchasing gifts for anniversaries, birthdays, Christmas/Holiday season, and Valentine's day.*
- ♥ *Optional romance includes big and little surprises, romantic dinners and dates, get-aways, sending flowers and/or cards, love letters, massages, and romantic movies.*

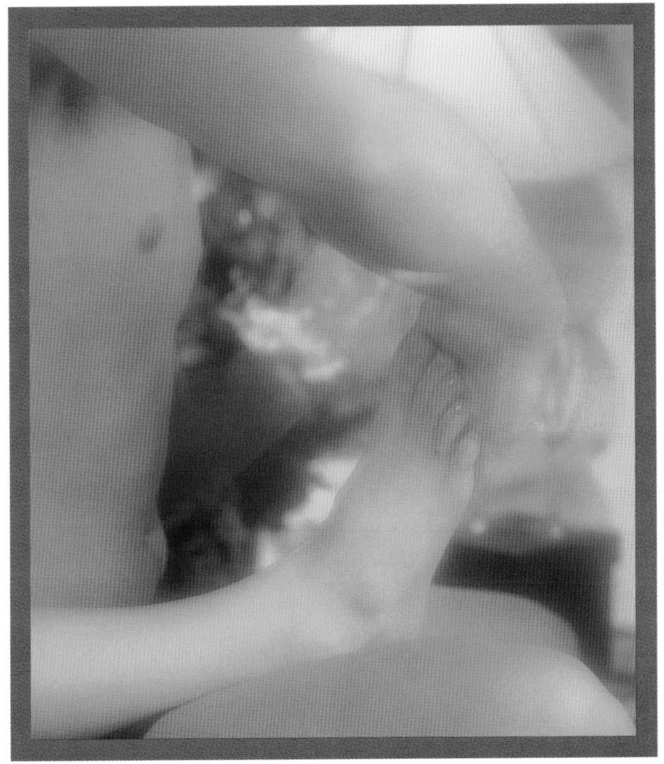

Romance does not have to be confined to weekends. Weekend romance may be more leisurely and planned, but weekday romance can be more spontaneous, impulsive, and bring out the unexpected.

7 After sliding between the toes, use your fingertips to lightly tap the top and sides of the foot from the toes to the ankle and back for a minute or two. This stroke feels like rain drops.

7a Next, turn your attention to the bottom of the foot. Use a light whipping action with the tips of your fingers. Whip the foot bottom from heel to toes. This is a stimulating and playful stroke.

8 Finally, finish the foot with light effleurage strokes. Use both hands to glide half way up the leg and back again. On the way down, separate your hands to stroke the top and bottom of the foot. Repeat several times moving slower with each stroke. End with a hold. Repeat massage strokes on the other foot.

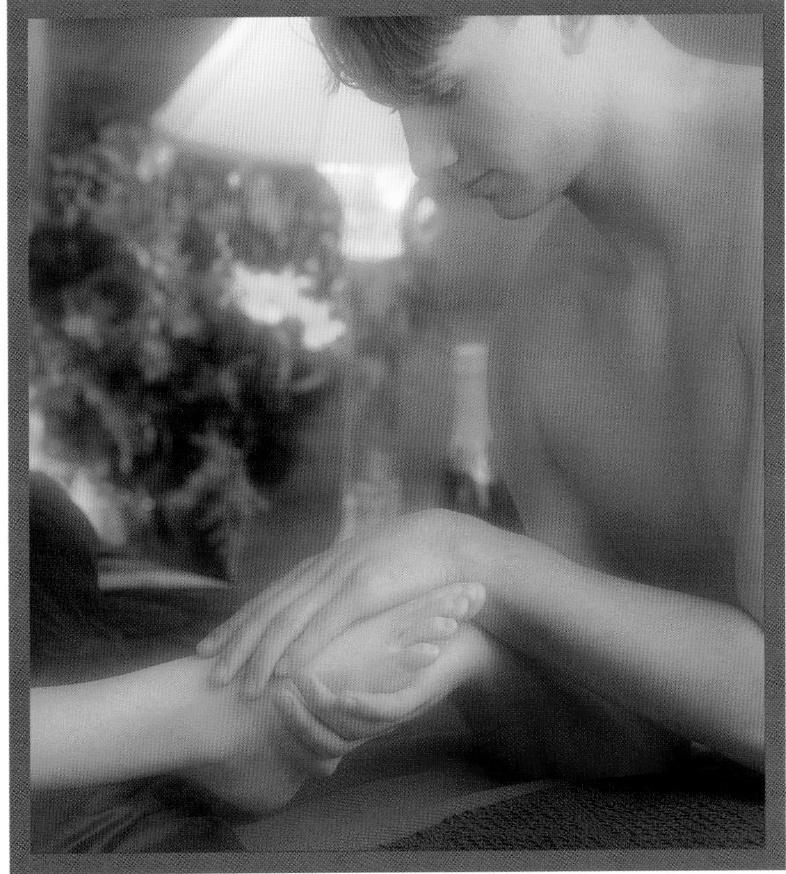

♥ *"Healthy loving is setting priorities in your life so there is time to create a safe, intimate, and beautiful environment for the ongoing discovery of each other."*

♥ *"Healthy loving is recognizing the need for playfulness, spontaneity, and the pleasuring of each other, thus providing treasured moments that nurture, encourage, and support the relationship."*

Jacqui Stratton and Susan Lawton

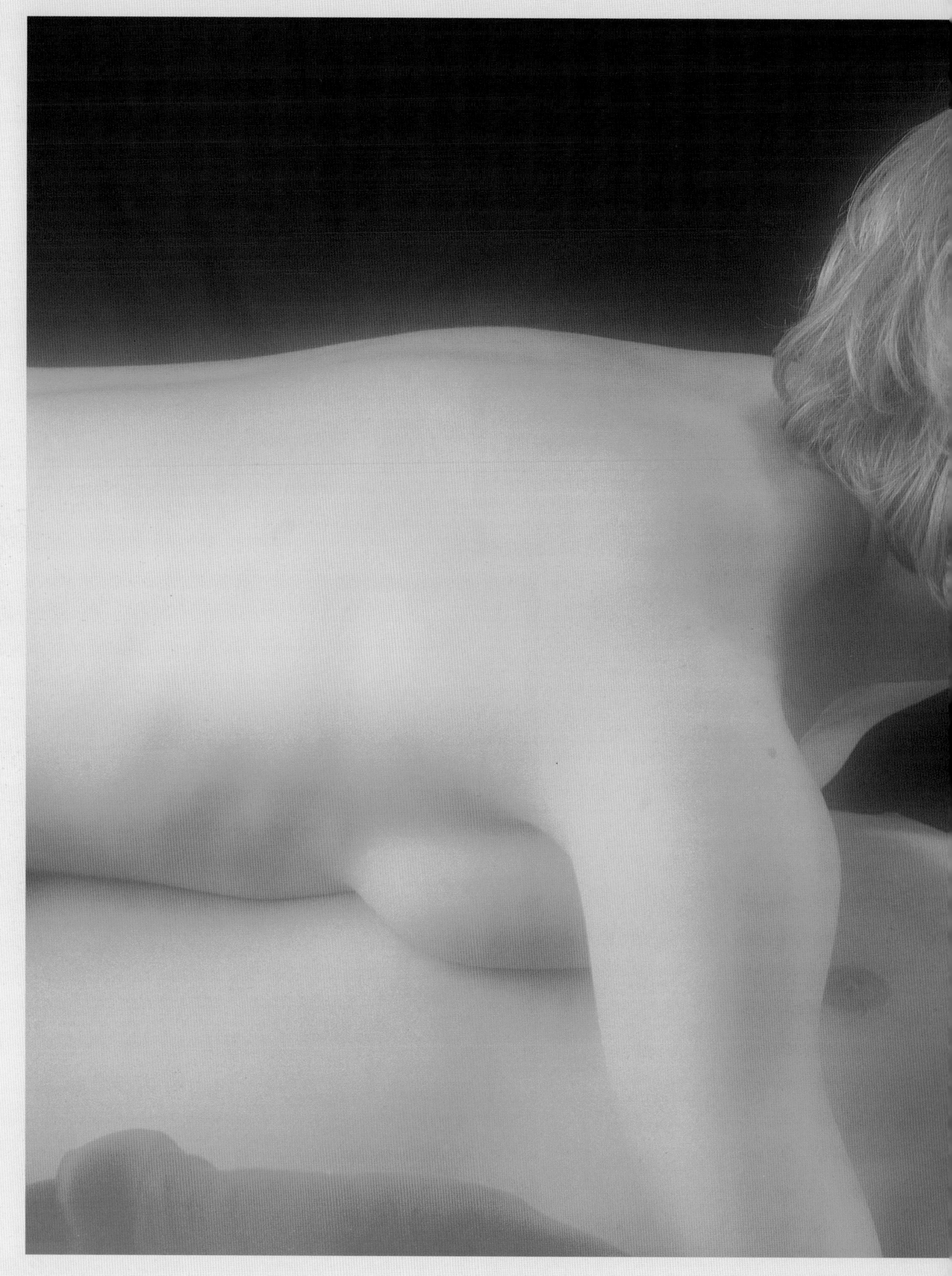

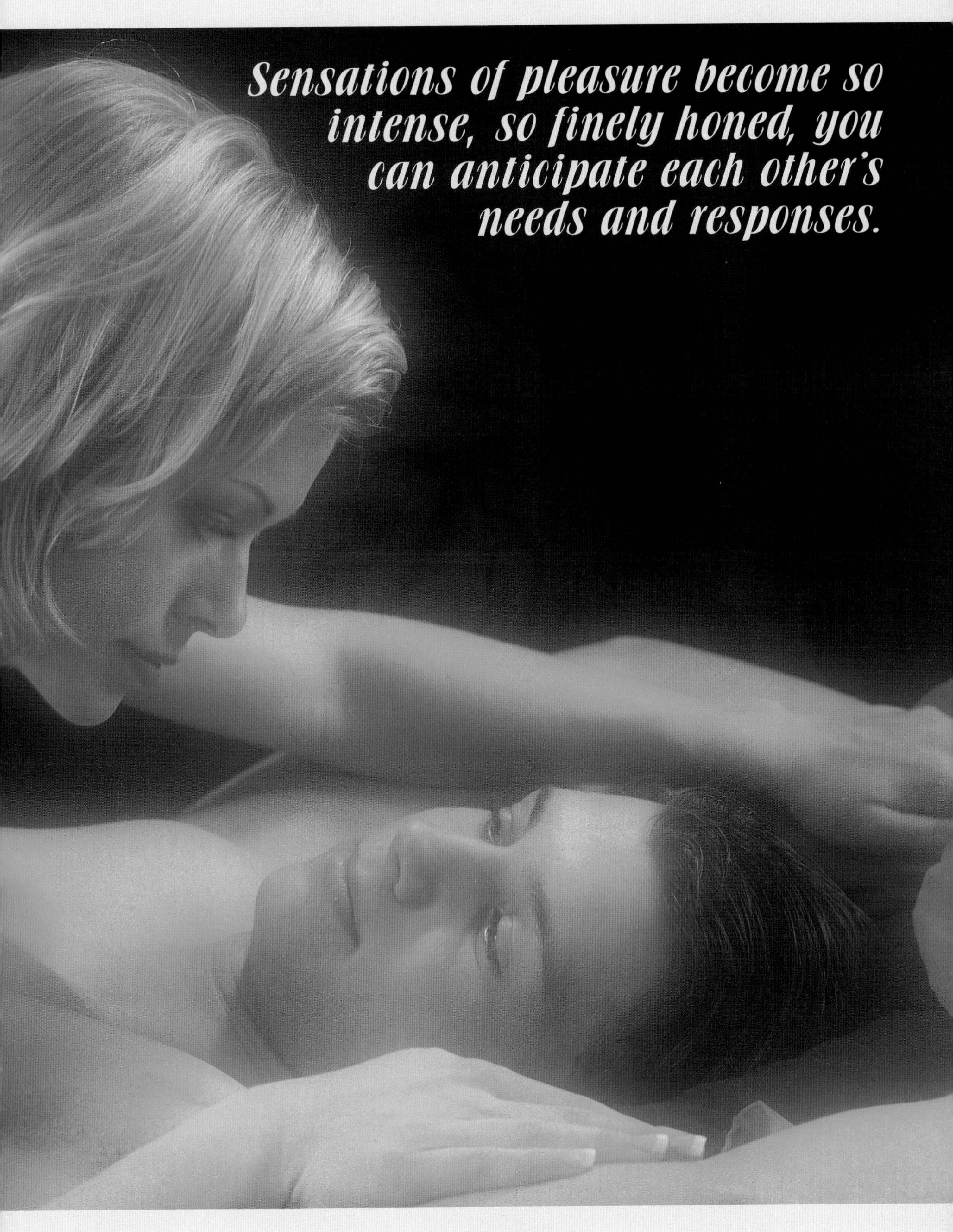
Sensations of pleasure become so intense, so finely honed, you can anticipate each other's needs and responses.

chapter seven

Continued Pleasures

If your lover thought romantic massage couldn't get much better than that incredible foot rub, they should think again. The front side of the body has more free nerve endings than the back side. In addition, the front of the body is more vulnerable. After all, this is where vital organs can be directly accessed. This is where emotions, loves, and insecurities lie; and, with increased awareness and increased protection comes increased sensitivity and sensation. If you — as the massage giver — are perceptive to your lover's needs and desires, they will be responsive to your acutely sensitive touch.

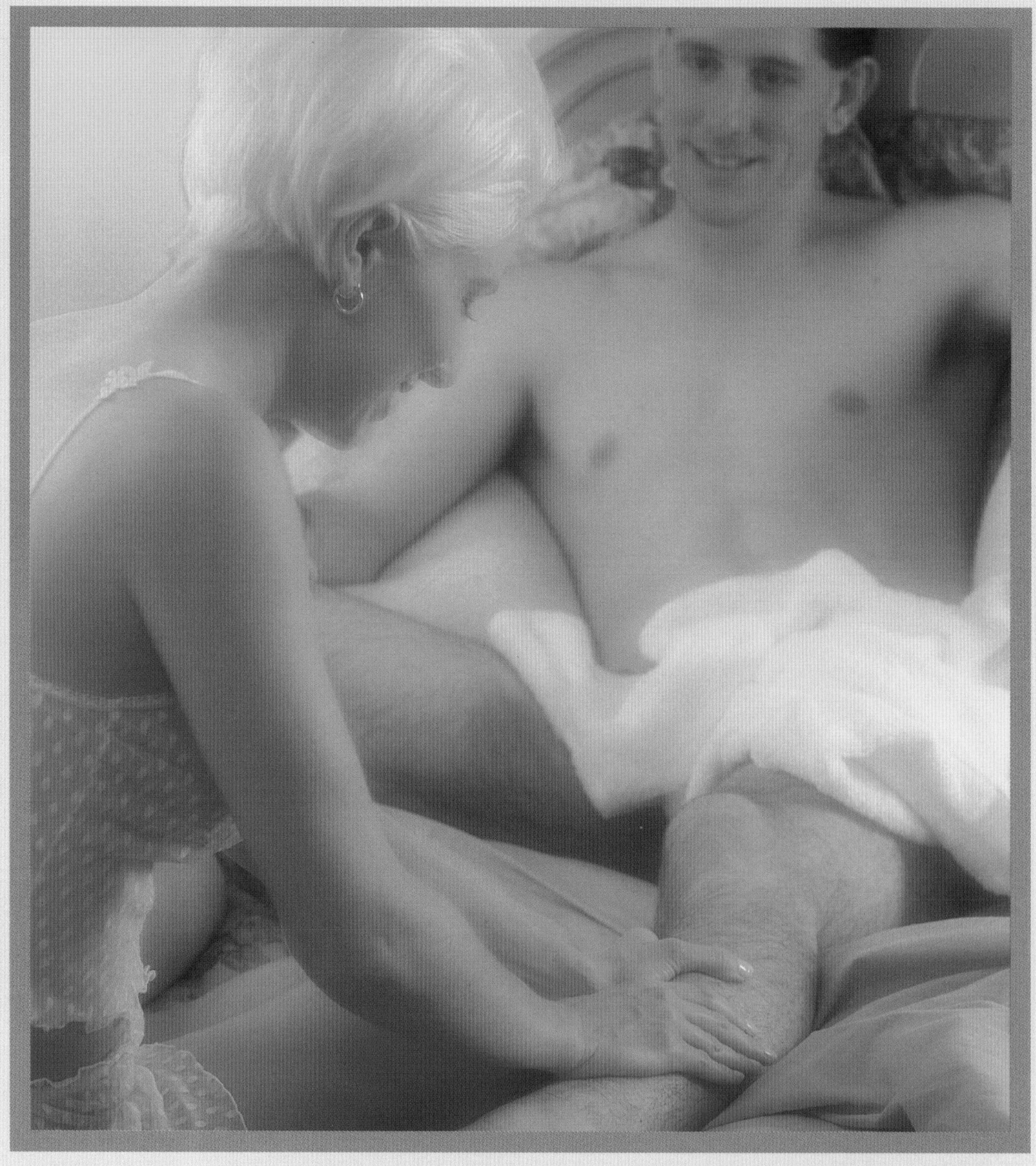

Front Leg & Thigh

Prior to massaging the front leg and thigh, determine whether there is minimal body hair. The less leg hair, the less oil needed to lubricate the skin. The more hair, the more oil required to lessen friction.

1 Make certain the legs are separated sufficiently to allow you access up the thigh. Place your hand just above the ankle. Pour oil on top of your hand and, with your free hand, scoop up the extra oil and begin spreading it up the leg slowly, using light effleurage strokes. As you need more oil, apply it to the top of your hand as it moves slowly. By applying oil "on-the-run," your partner will not be distracted by the stop and start action massage can take when someone halts abruptly to add oil to skin. Continue applying oil up the leg and thigh to the top of the hip. Make deep flowing strokes up and return lightly.

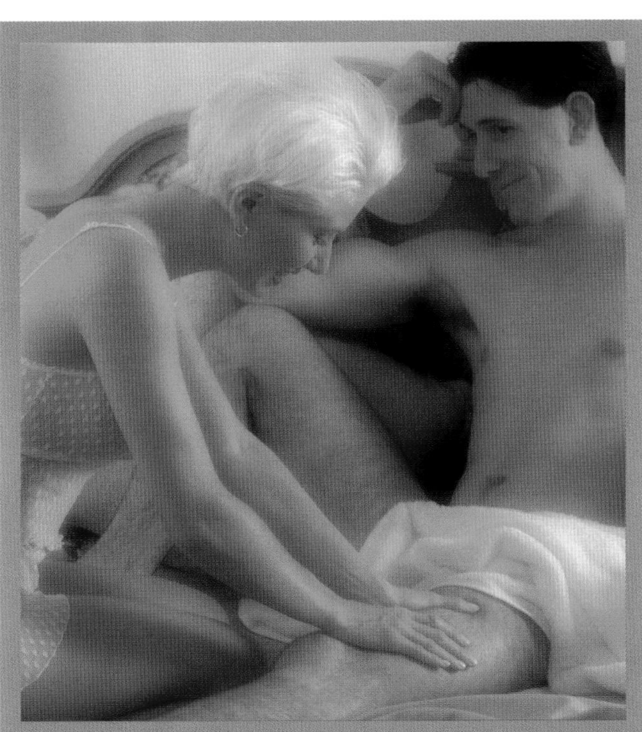

2 Begin kneading the fleshy inner portion of the leg with the heel of your thumb. Then, as you position yourself to the side, and pull your partner's leg muscles, alternate a back and forth motion with either hand. Repeat this stroke for several minutes, moving up and down the leg.

2a Continue this same stroke moving up the leg to the kneecap. Slide one hand up the leg over the kneecap to grasp the flesh above it. Slide the other hand down the thigh over the kneecap to grasp the flesh below it. Repeat this for a minute or two.

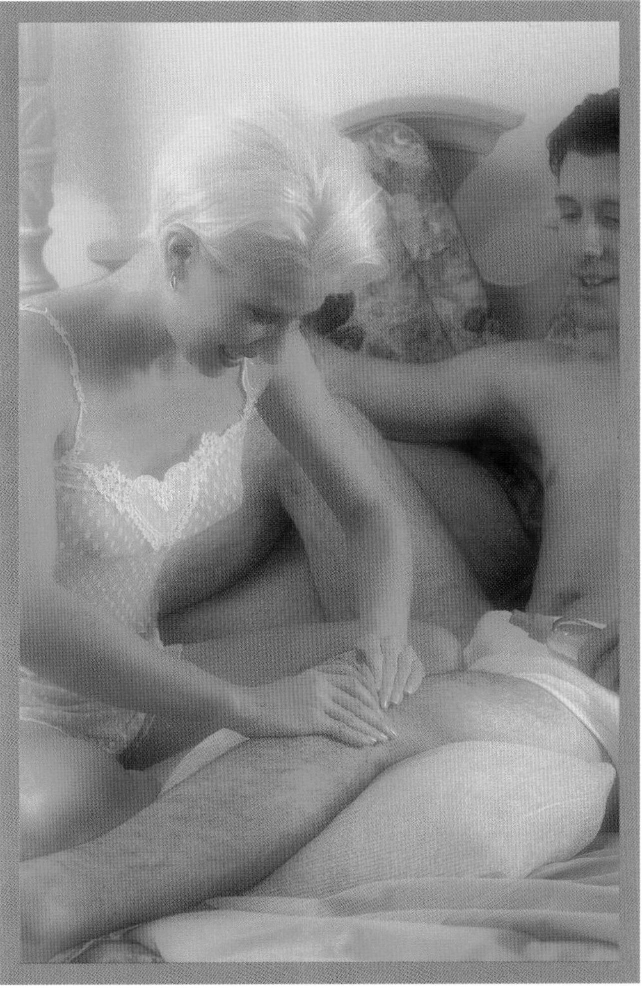

Certain talismans or charms are believed to bring luck to love. Hearts, the most common, mean constancy and joy. Blue "eye" beads (in the shape of an eye) promote love affairs. The fish is an ancient Egyptian charm for domestic happiness. Frogs are from the Romans and ensure mutual ardor and happy relationships. Keys, a Japanese talisman, bring love, wealth, and general happiness.

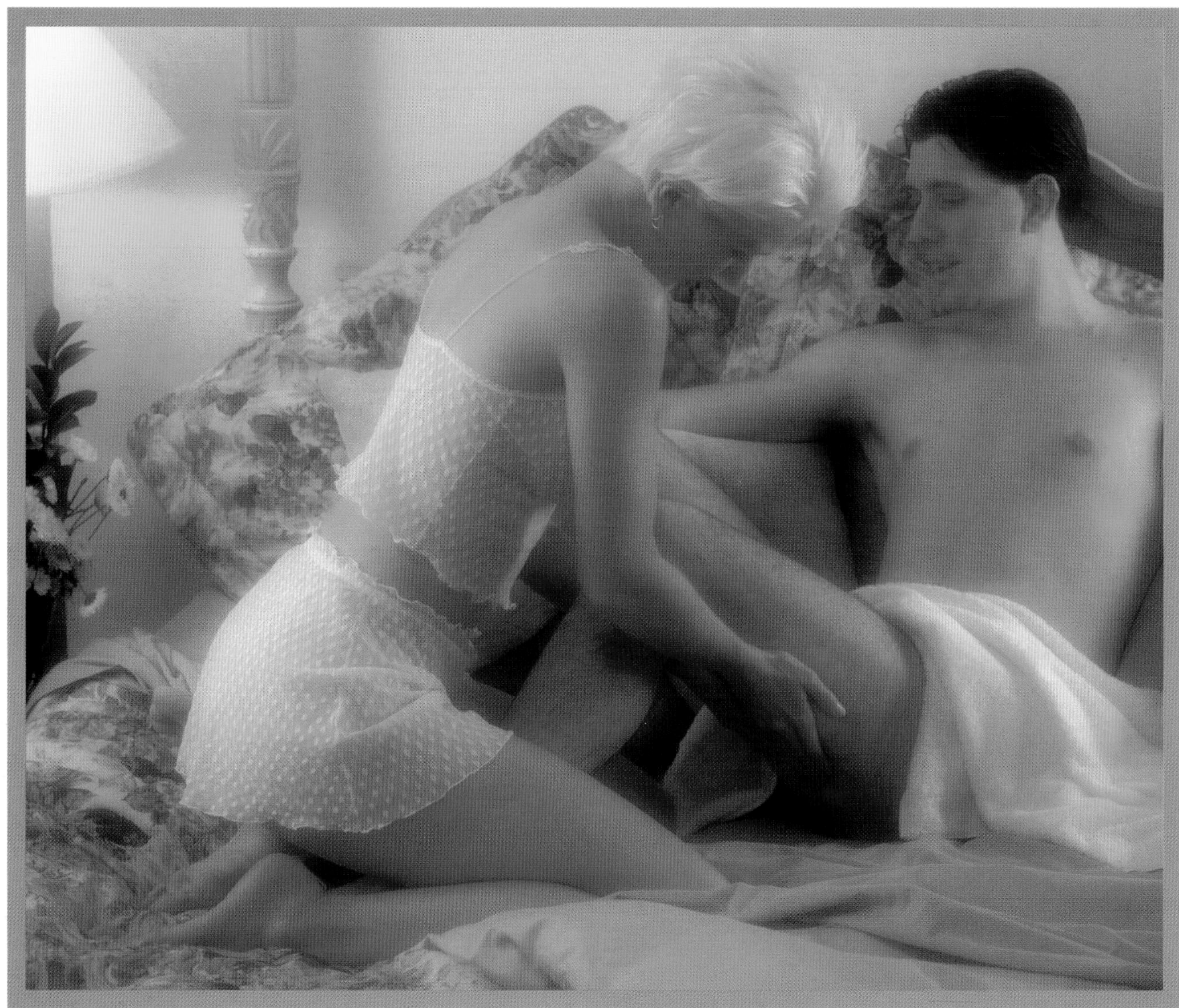

3 Once you have completed kneading the thigh, bend the leg straight up at the knee. Prop the knee on your stomach. From this position, you can address both the leg and the thigh. Use deep effleurage with overlapping thumbs or straight knuckles to iron as you massage toward the hip. Return lightly with open hands and relaxed fingers. Make this return stroke slow; linger at the inner thigh using a feathering technique. This is an exquisitely erotic touch that will arouse feelings of desire for you as you massage close to the genitals. Repeat this sequence for several minutes. If you should happen to brush up against their genitals, watch their face for expressions of acceptance and satisfaction. If not, this is not the right time; avoid any genital contact for now.

3a To add variety to this deep effleurage stroke of the thigh and the leg, place both hands under the thigh near the buttock and lift up in a slow and even stroke up the back of the thigh. This stroke utilizes your lover's natural body weight and gravity to create deep pressure as you lift up and allow your hands to gently glide up the back of the thigh toward the back of the knee. Ease off pressure as you approach the back of the knee to avoid causing any discomfort. Repeat this stroke or blend it with the deep ironing with knuckles for several minutes.

3b Place one hand behind the knee and lower the leg down with the other hand when done.

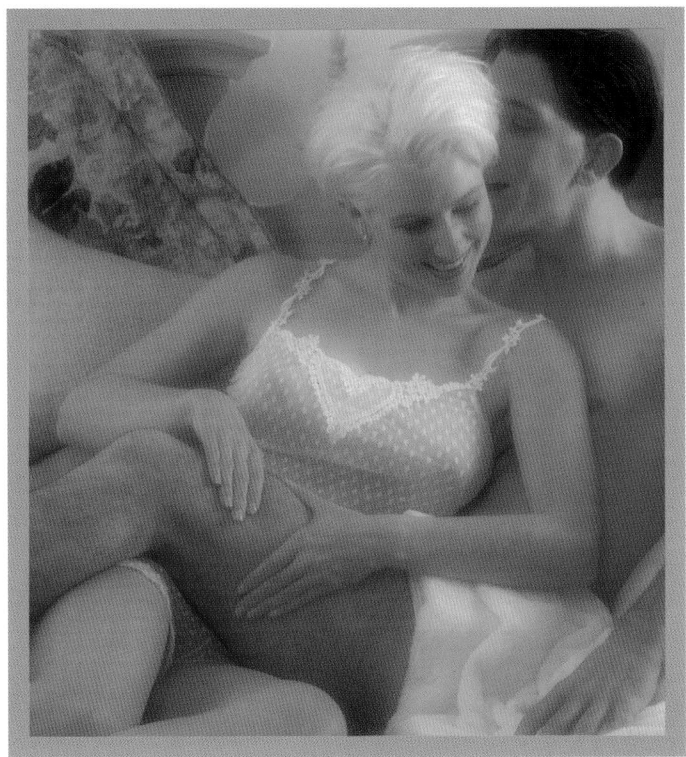

4 With your partner's leg now fully extended, begin cross fiber massage of the thigh. Place one hand firmly at the inner thigh; the other on the outer thigh. Push and pull together with your hands passing within several inches of each other. Now, go back again. Repeat this stroke from just above the knee up to the groin and back several times. Remember the inner thigh is a sensitive area. You can massage deeply, just move slowly The deeper you go, the slower the stroke.

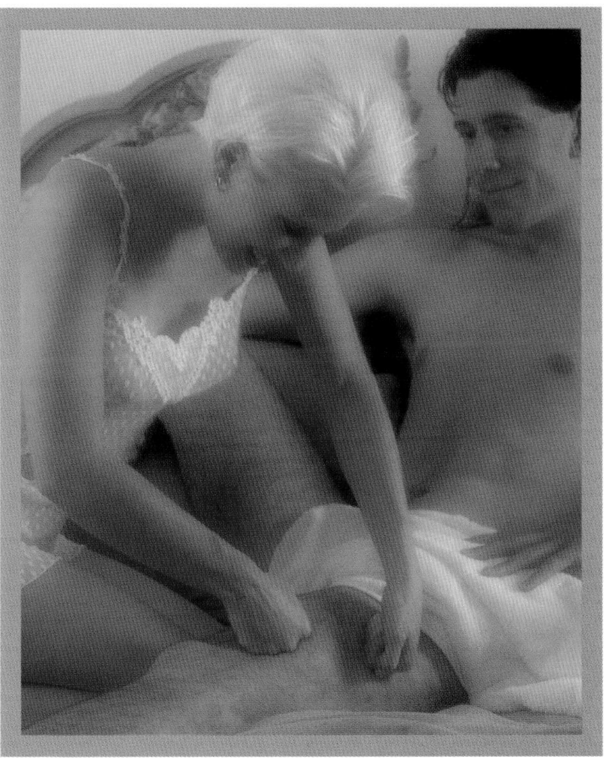

"O, my luve is like a red, red rose,
That's newly sprung in June.
O, my luve is like the melodie,
That's sweetly played in tune.

As fair art thou, my bonnie lass,
So deep in luve am I,
And I will luve thee still, my dear,
While the sands o' life shall run.

Till a' the seas gang dry, my dear,
and the rocks melt wi' the sun!
And I will luve thee still, my dear,
While the sands o' life shall run.

And fare thee well, my only luve,
And faire thee weel awhile!
And I will come again, my luve,
Though it were ten thousand mile!"
Robert Burns

5 Now try deep friction to the thigh muscles along their fiber orientation. Place one hand at the inner thigh just above the knee, the other hand at the outer hip joint. Do this cross fiber push pull technique only lengthwise along the muscles. Again, allow the hands to pass within several inches of each other. As you continue this back and forth movement, try to go deeper and faster. This creates friction, which increases deep heating action on this large muscle. It feels like someone turned on a heating pad. The heat helps relax those muscles. Repeat for a minute or two.

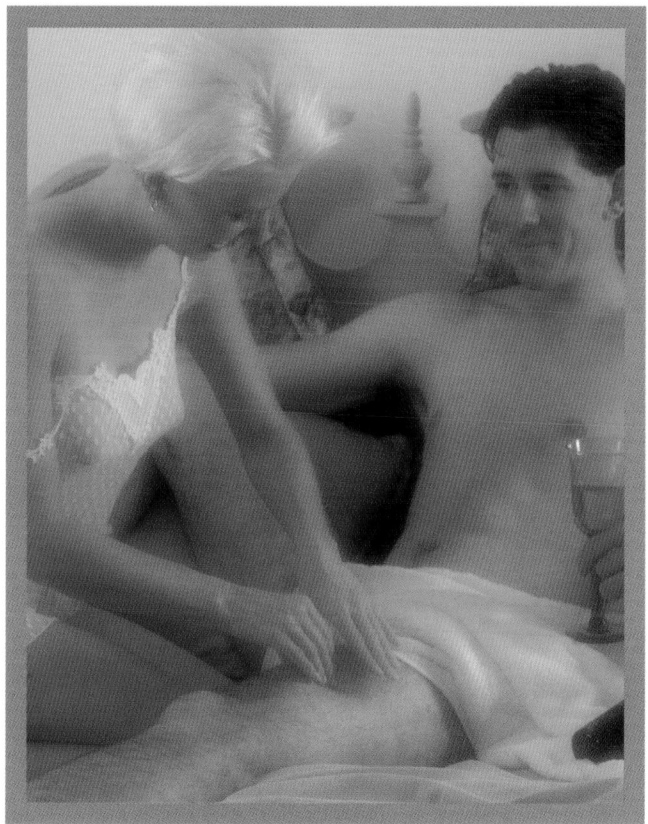

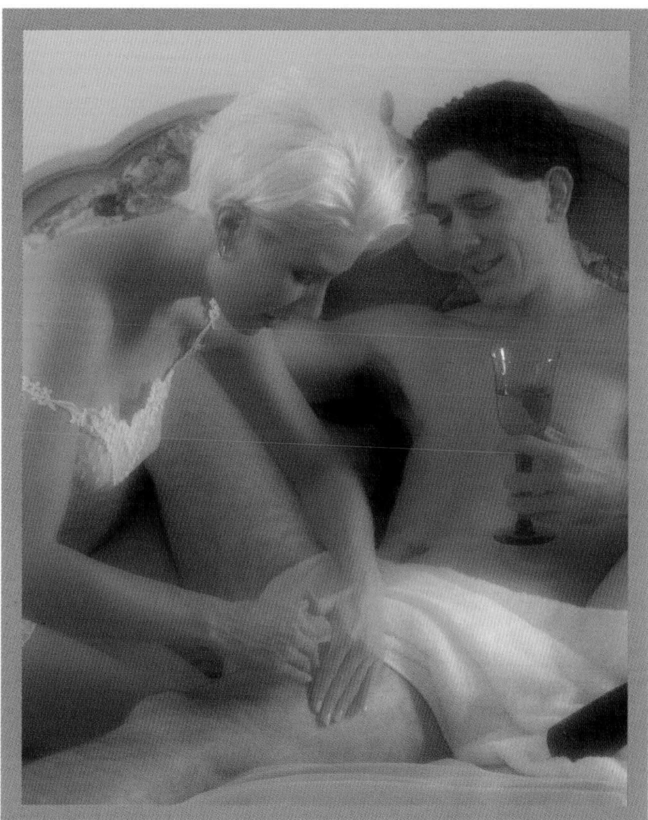

6 Before ending the effleurage stroke, try some stimulating percussive strokes. Blend plucking of the leg and thigh with whipping and hacking. By alternating between these three strokes, you can continue this teasingly aggressive massage until your partner's skin starts to visually glow and become flushed. This is an indication that blood is near the surface and circulation is improving. Do not use hacking on bony sections like the kneecap or shinbone, but you can stroke the inner thigh. Use light pressure so you do not irritate the skin. You want to increase your partner's touch awareness toward the goal of heightened passion, not destroy your chances for romance by hurting them in this sensitive place.

"You're never too old ... You're never too sophisticated ... You're never too independent ... You're never too cool ... You've never had so much therapy ... that you won't benefit from a little romance."

Gregory J.P. Godek, "1001 More Ways To Be Romantic"

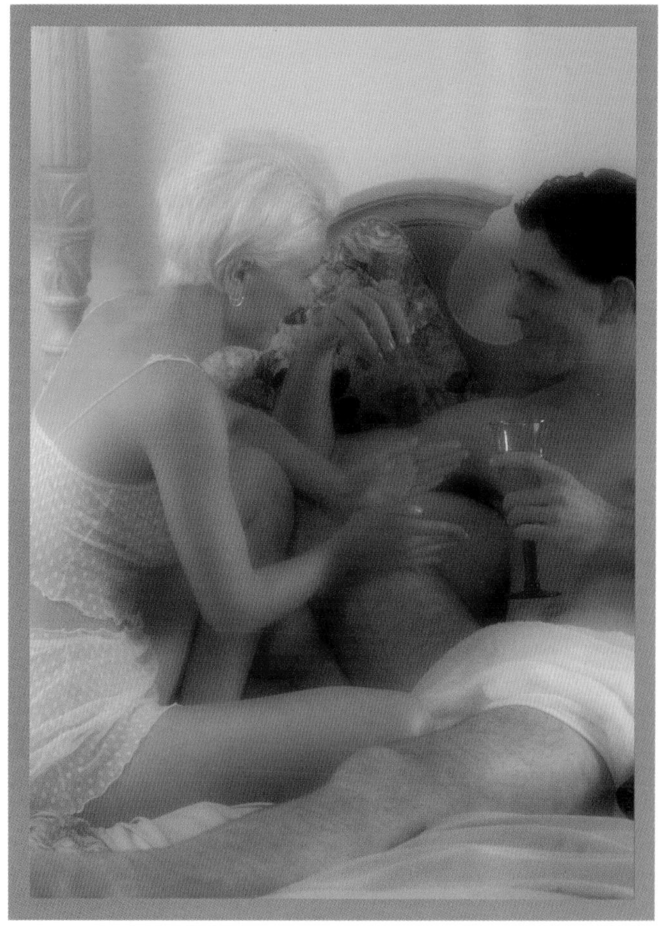

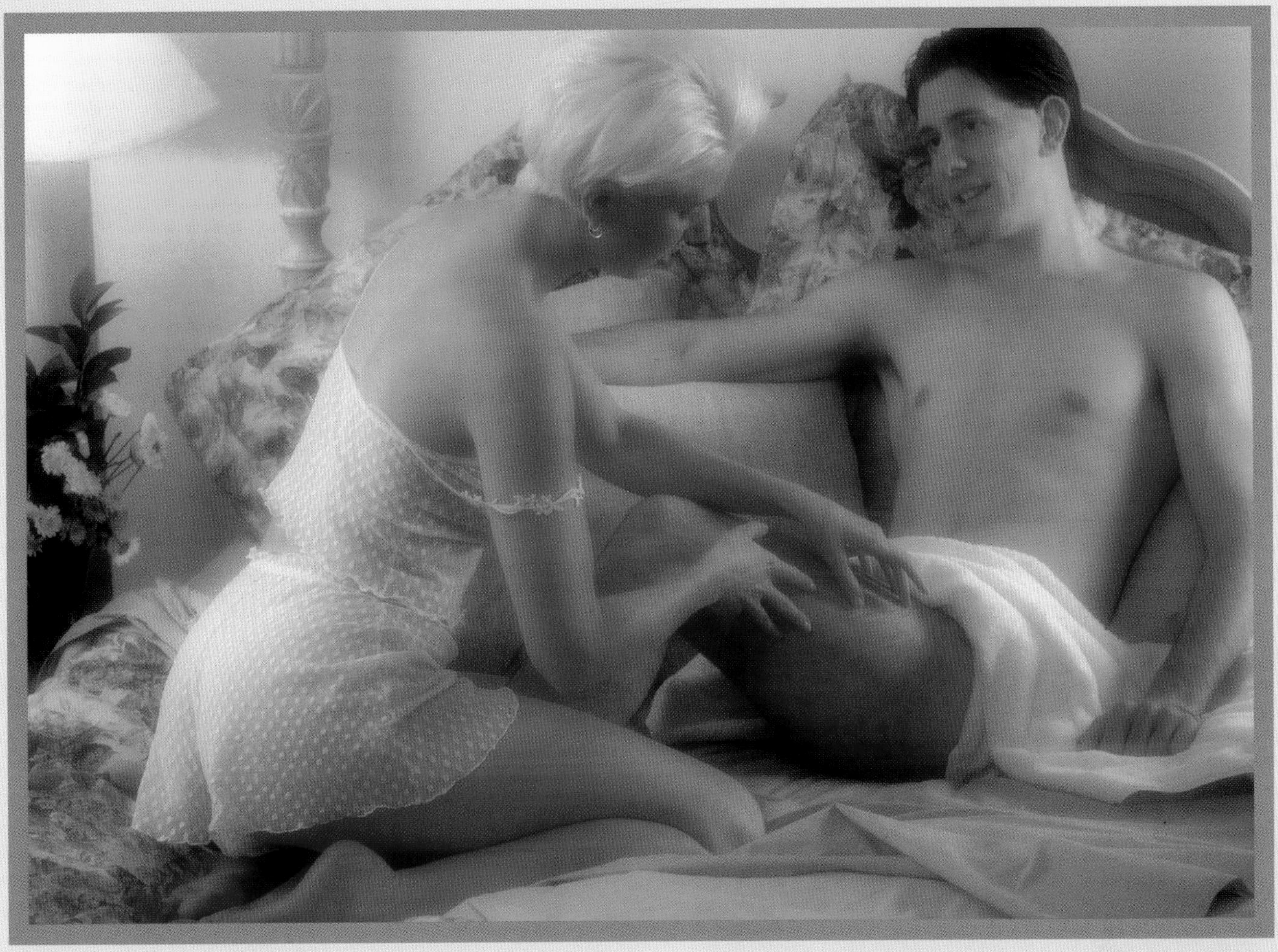

7 End by soothing the muscles using light effleurage up the leg and thigh to the hip bone. Allow your hands to separate, with one going down the outside of the leg and the other gliding down the groin and inner thigh. Use a feathering technique or just let your fingers linger between your lover's thigh — caressing it, brushing it, enticing them to desire this type of touch. This is a major erogenous zone that arouses sexual feelings in your lover. If you happen to brush up against the genitals or pubic hair ever so lightly, it can stimulate their interest and ignite their desires for you in intimate ways. Repeat this entire set of strokes on the other leg.

8 When you have finished working both legs, hold both legs above the ankles and lift several inches and gently traction (pull) the legs. Then let the legs rest.

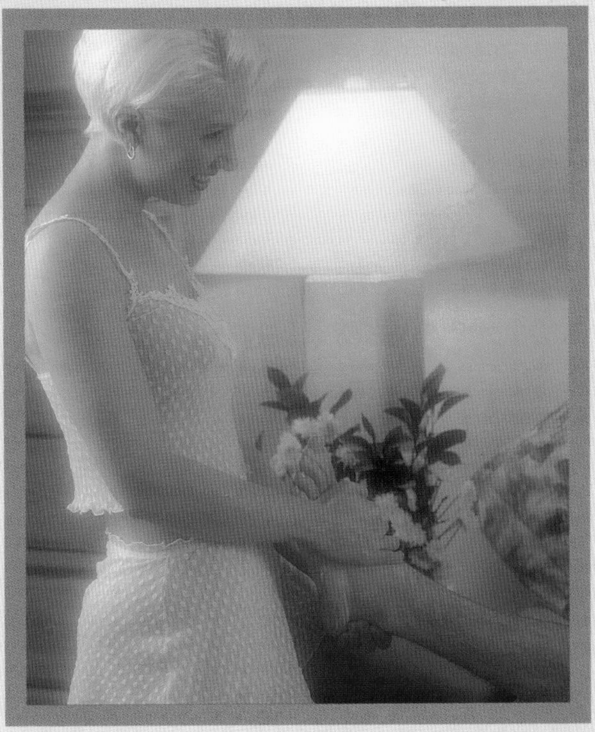

Arms & Hands

1 Turn your attention to the arms. Apply sufficient oil to coat the arm, the lubrication will reduce friction. Remember more hair on the arms means more oil, less hair less oil. Massage along the length of the arm; use both hands to spread oil from the wrist to the shoulder joint. Begin one hand at the shoulder and the other hand at the wrist. Do the push pull stroke allowing both hands to pass within an inch or two of each other. If you push with both hands starting at the wrist, you will shove the shoulder until it is uncomfortably hunched up.

1a Now lift the arm to bend at the elbow and massage with effleurage from wrist to elbow joint and return lightly. Alternate, using both hands to effleurage down the arm. This allows muscles to be massaged on both sides of the arm.

2 Hold the hand so your thumbs are in the palm of your partner's hand, and your fingers are opposite the palm. Use petrissage movements with your thumbs to squeeze and tease as you work the muscles. Be certain not to bend their wrist too much one way or the other. Repeat this for several minutes.

> *"While the foundation of romance is a serious love, the nature of romance is lighthearted."*
> *Author Unknown*

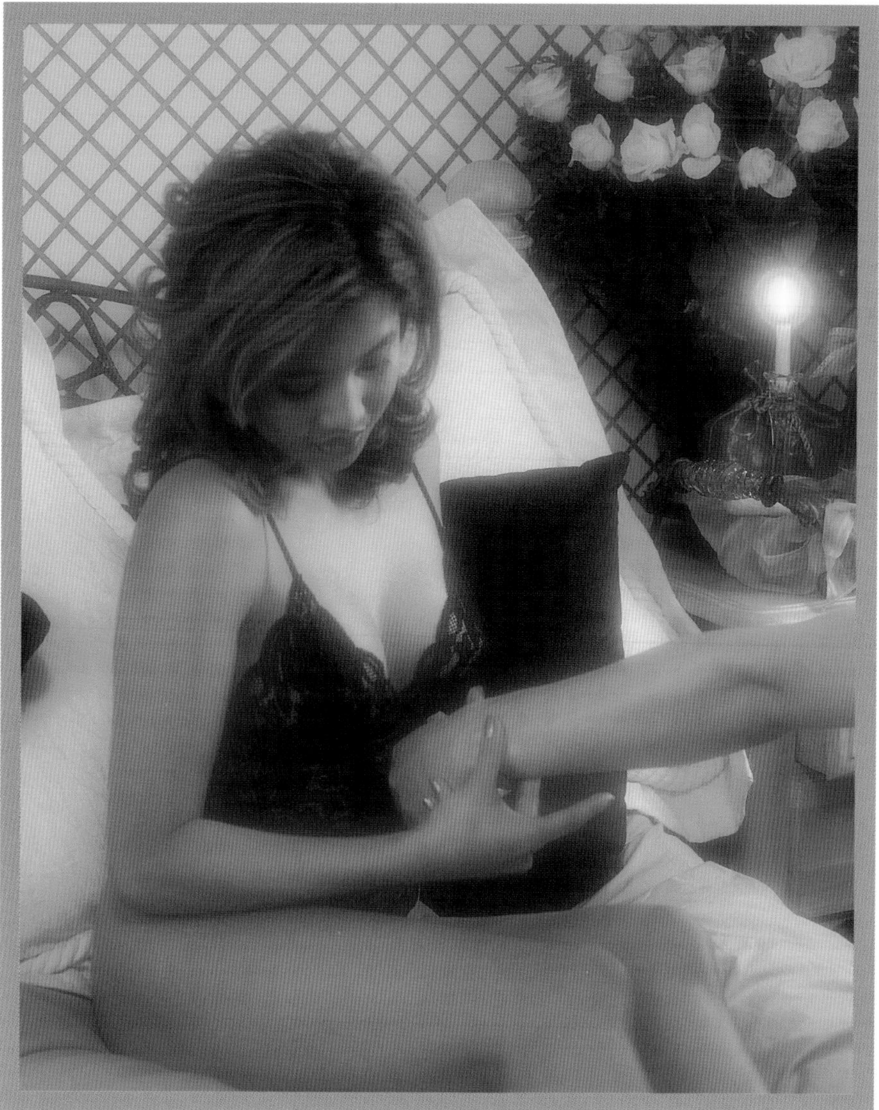

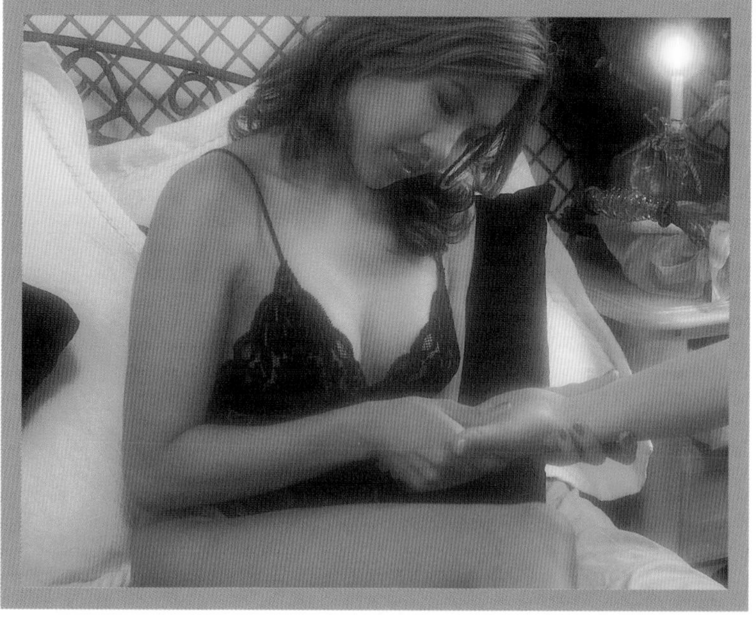

3 Now massage the fingers. Support the wrist with one hand as you start at the base of the thumb and slowly, and firmly slide upward making a slow, and deliberate cork screw motion up to the tip of the thumb. Repeat each finger three times, moving slower each time you repeat. Because of the large amount of nerves in each finger tip, this playful massaging brings pleasurable smiles to your partner's face.

3a You may even do what's called a finger "snap." Grasp a finger between your index and middle fingers and pull lightly but aggressively all the way to the tip of their finger. The stroke makes a snapping sound as your index and middle fingers strike each other at the end of the motion.

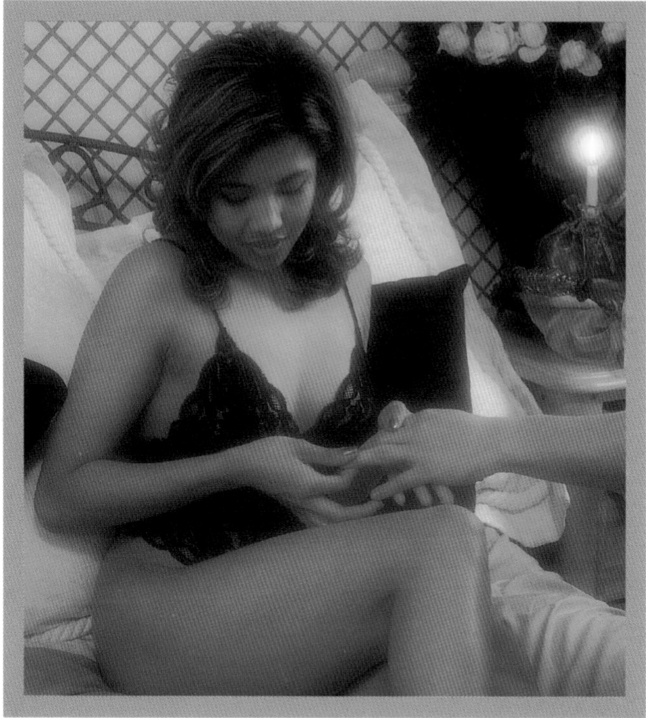

Send a message with flowers:

Apple blossom	*preference*
Camellia, white	*perfected loveliness*
Carnation	*pure love*
Chrysanthemum, white	*truth*
Cornflower	*hope*
Daffodil	*regard*
Daisy	*innocence*
Fern	*fascination*
Forget-me-not	*true love*
Gardenia	*secret untold love*
Geranium, oak leafed	*true friendship*
Geranium, rose scented	*preference*
Hydrangea	*boasting*
Jasmine	*amiability*
Iris	*message*
Lilac	*first love*
Myrtle	*love*
Pansy	*love, courtship*
Rose	*love*
Sweet pea	*pleasure*
Tulip, red	*declaration of love*
Violet	*faithfulness*

4 Next, take both hands and grasp the thumb and index finger knuckles at their base with your thumb and opposing fingers. Make small rotating motions to help relieve tension in the tendons and ligaments between the knuckles. Do this rotation for five seconds, and then move on to the index and middle finger knuckles, and so on.

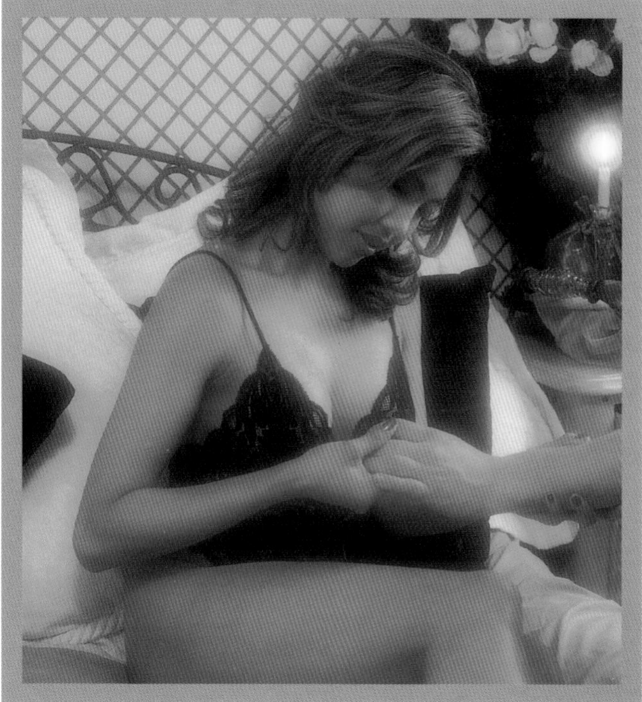

5 After rotating the fingers, hold your partner's hand with one of your hands while your other hand grasps just above their wrist joint. Keeping the arm above the wrist stable, rotate the hand in slow circles. This gives the wrist joint, and all of the wrist bones and their ligaments a chance to release tension stored there from on the job or repetitive stress. Do this for five seconds.

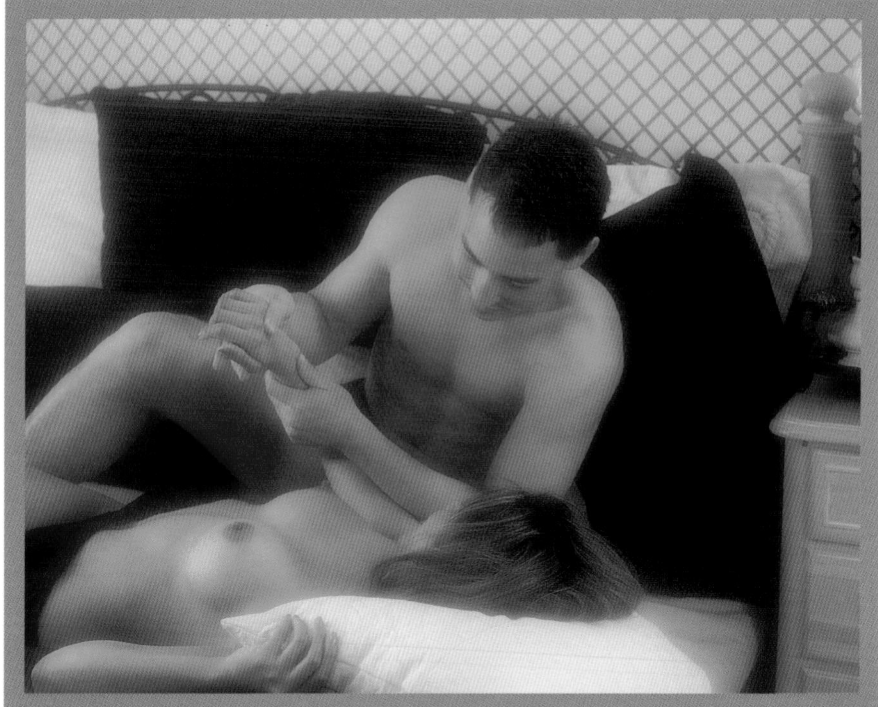

6 When finished rotating the wrist, extend the entire arm up and to the side of your partner's head. This exposes their upper arm with its powerful bicep and tricep muscles. Apply oil to your hands and briefly lubricate the upper arm with gliding strokes. Once lubricated, begin kneading the muscles. One hand should work the biceps while the other works the triceps. Continue this stroke for a minute or two.

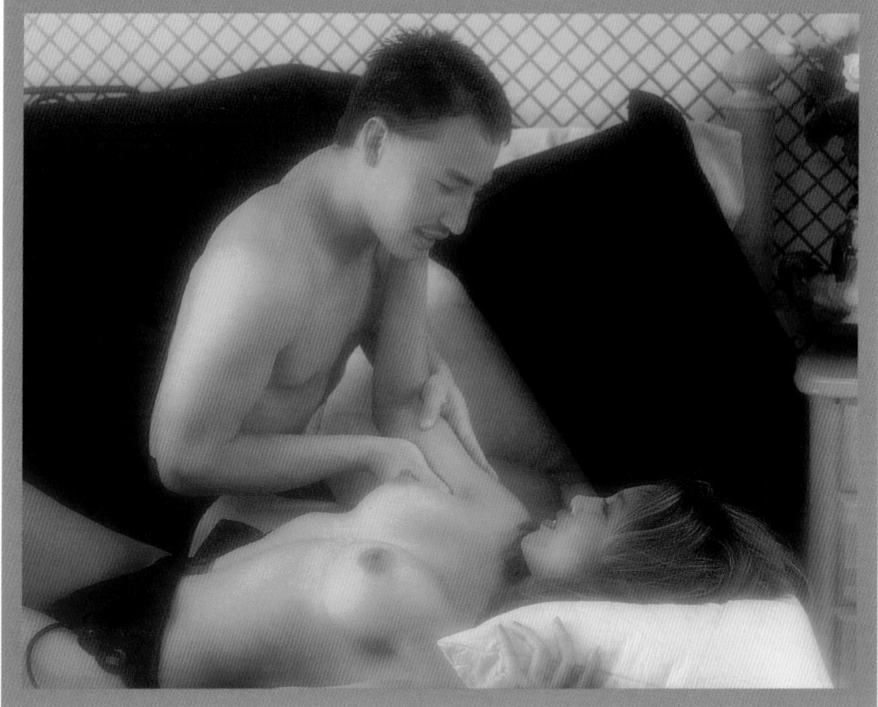

Ambiance is an important part of a Romantic Massage. If you are using background music to set the mood; you may want to take into consideration the use of a continuous-play tape player or a CD player that plays multiple CDs, so you do not have to get up to turn over a tape or change a CD.

7 Now, lift the upper arm, gripping the forearm side of the elbow joint with one hand. Massage the upper arm with your free hand using effleurage strokes. Extend the effleurage stroke from the upper arm, past the armpit and down the side of the body, as far as is comfortable for you. At the same time you are performing this stroke, slightly stretch the arm with your other hand. This stroke feels absolutely wonderful as your lover's torso is gently tractioned while being rubbed. The return stroke should be a light feathering that lingers as you pass through the center of the armpit. This may be ticklish to your lover. If it is, try feathering to either side of the armpit. Do this combination of strokes several times. Leave the arm in the extended position for massaging the chest next.

7a Do not forget to do the entire series of arm and hand strokes on the opposite side. Apply oil to the arm from the wrist to the shoulder joint with effleurage strokes. Focus on deeper strokes to the forearm. Use circular friction to the palm of the hand. Corkscrew each finger and snap it. Rotate the knuckles, and then the wrist. Knead the upper arm. Lift and extend the upper arm as you incorporate long stretching effleurage strokes to the arm and side of the body. Leave the arm extended to the side of the head for massaging your lover's chest.

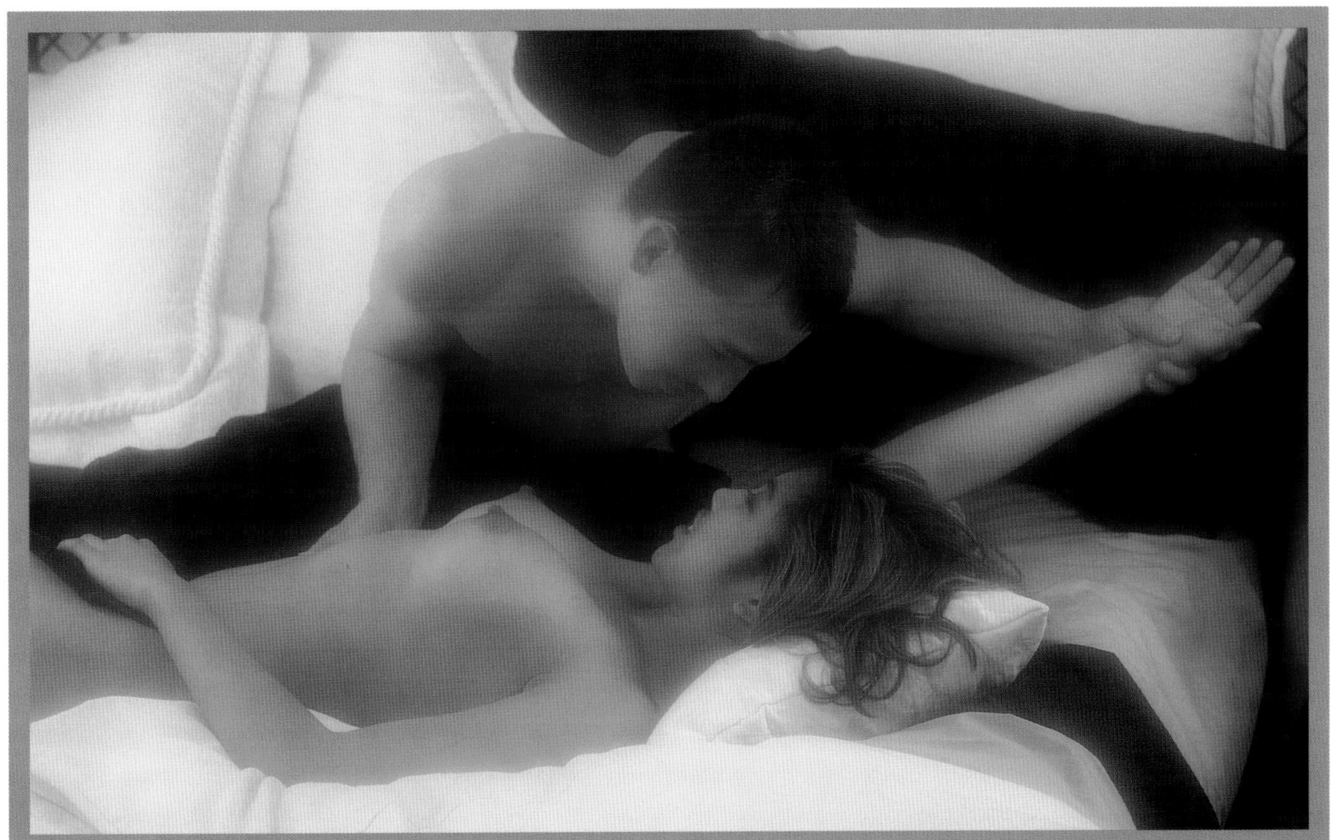

Some popular types and properties of carrier oils for massage:

- ♥ *Almond oil is the most popular with little smell, rich in protein, emollient, nourishing, and slow to become rancid.*
- ♥ *Apricot or peach kernel oils have the same properties as almond, but are more expensive.*
- ♥ *Grapeseed oil is very fine and clear and gives a satiny finish without feeling greasy.*
- ♥ *Hazelnut oil penetrates the easiest and deepest. It is stimulating to the circulation and nourishing to the skin.*
- ♥ *Jojoba oil gives a satiny feel and is slow to become rancid.*
- ♥ *Olive oil is calming, and relieves itching, but overpowering to the fragrance of essential oils.*

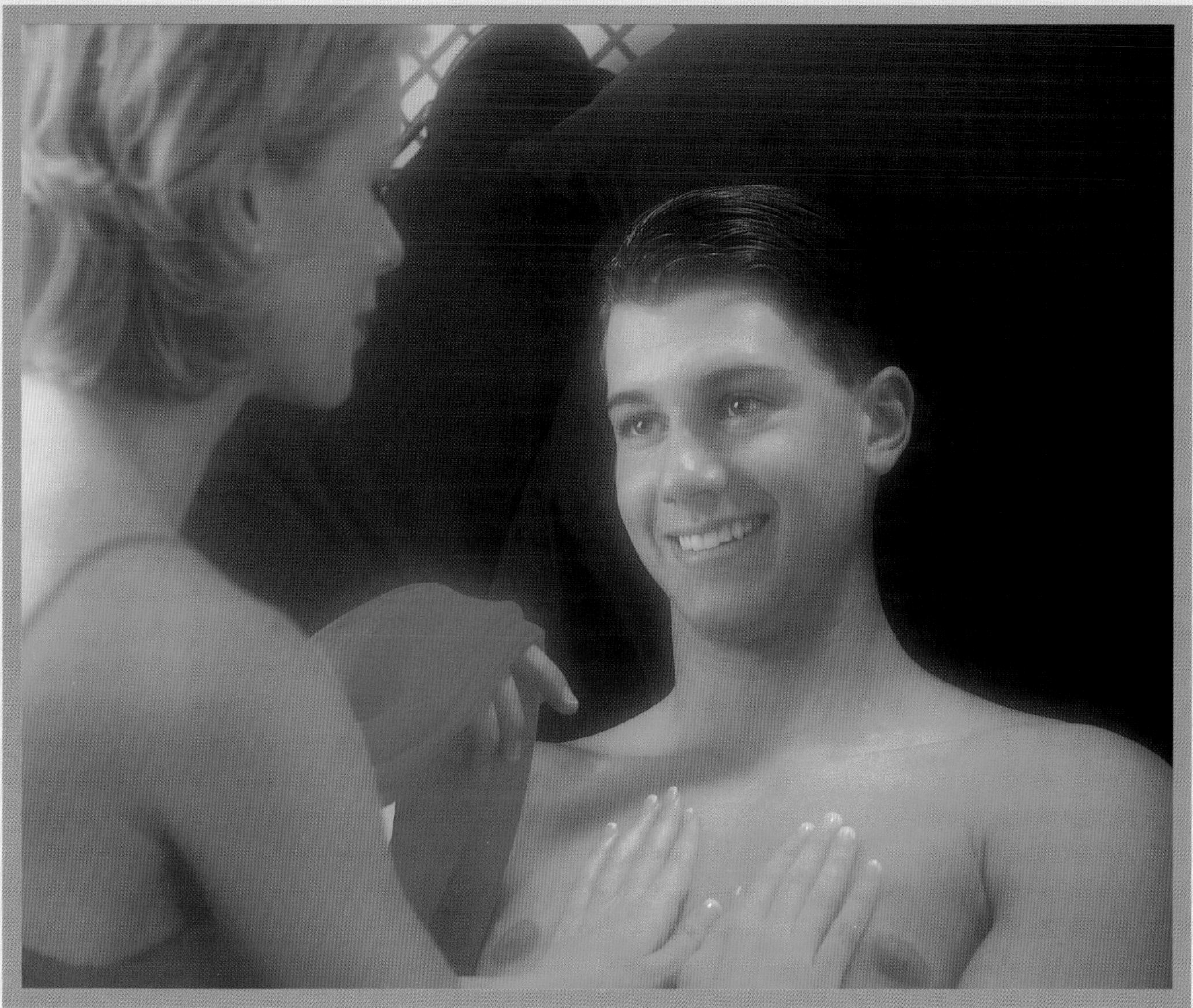

Chest & Abdomen

We have finally arrived at the portion of massage least understood — the chest. We are most vulnerable at this section of our body. We tend to protect that which is dearest to us. The chest represents our heart, our nurturing, our love, our openness, and our vulnerability; especially when we allow someone in to that space. As we shield ourselves from possible heartache and disappointments, pains and sorrows; we unconsciously hold tension in the muscles of the chest. If these holding patterns become chronic, if we hold these issues over long periods of time, our chest muscles need massage and relaxation.

1 Begin at your lover's side. Apply enough oil to the palm of your hand to lubricate the entire chest, abdomen, and sides. Start with a light effleurage stroke several inches below the breast bone. With your hands next to each other, move slowly up the chest between the nipples to the collar bone, where your hands will part and glide toward the shoulders, up past the armpit, and as far up the arm as you can comfortably go. Return with a light effleurage, over the armpit and down the sides to the abdomen. Bring your hands together and proceed to the breast bone to repeat the stroke again. You may repeat this six or more times, varying pressure and making the path of your stroke more broad.

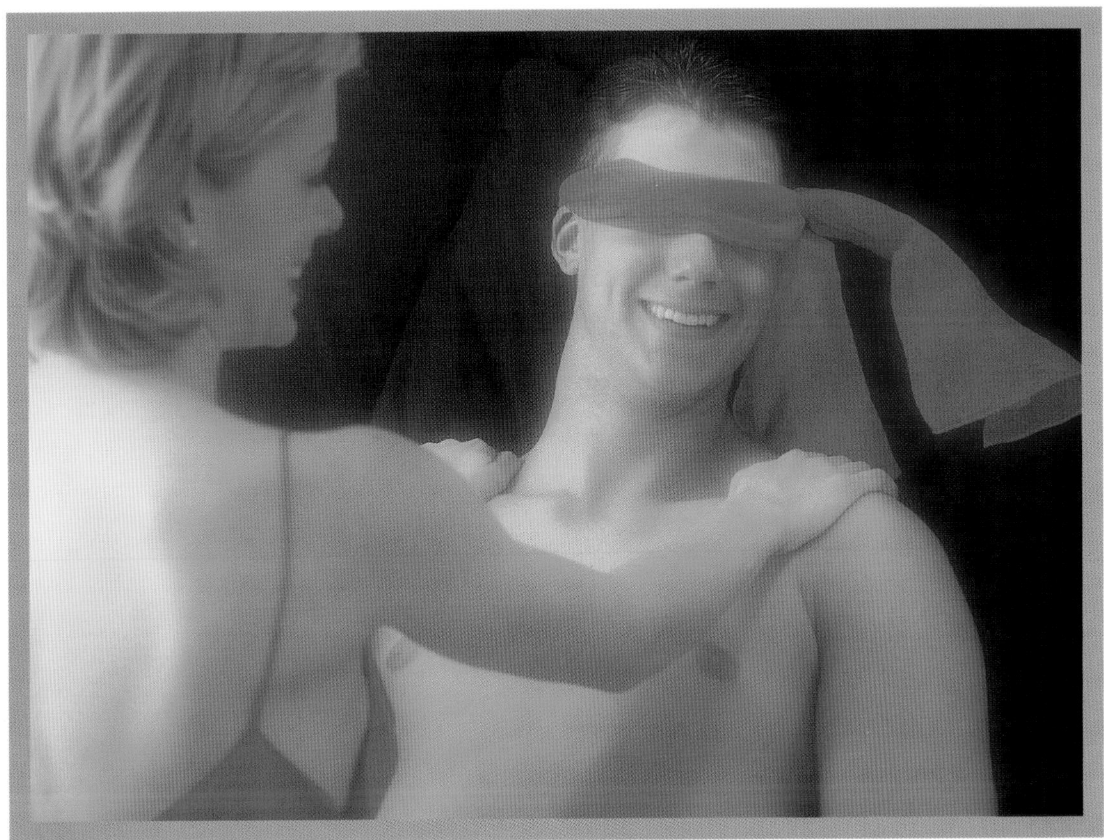

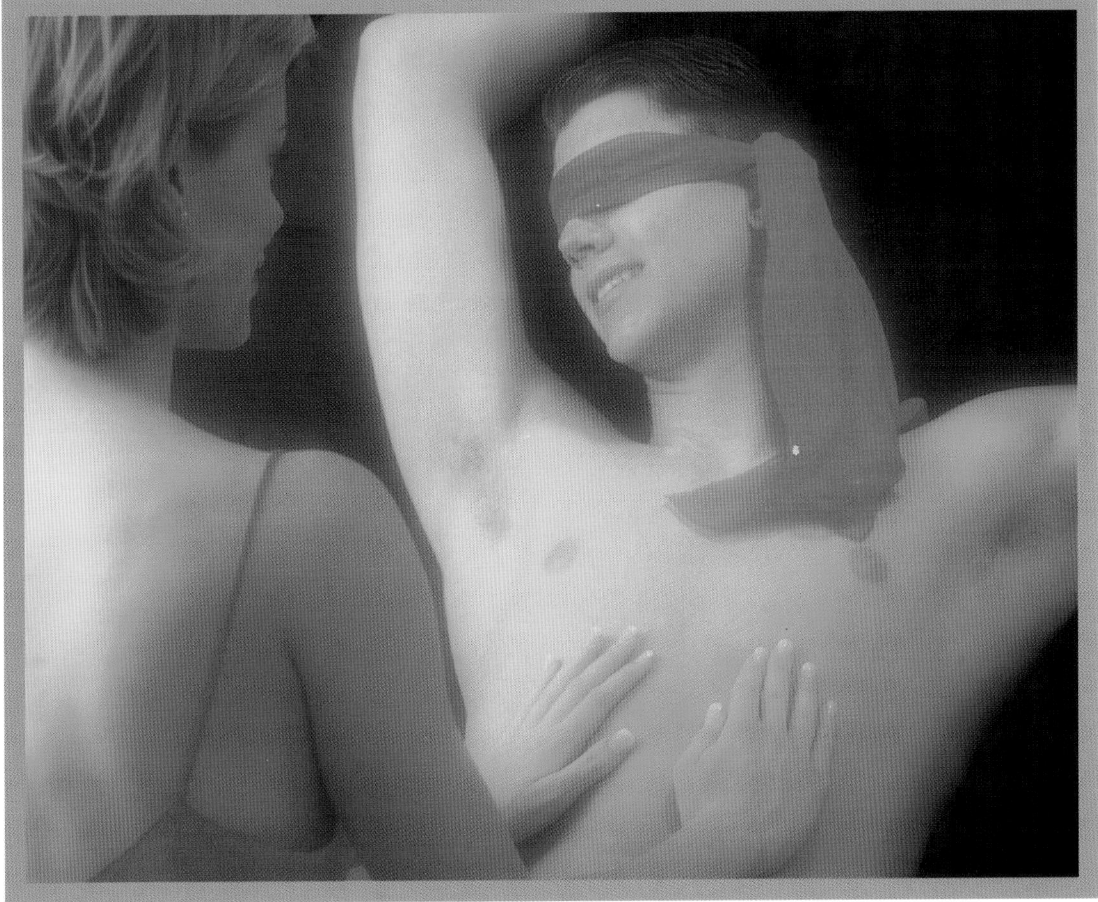

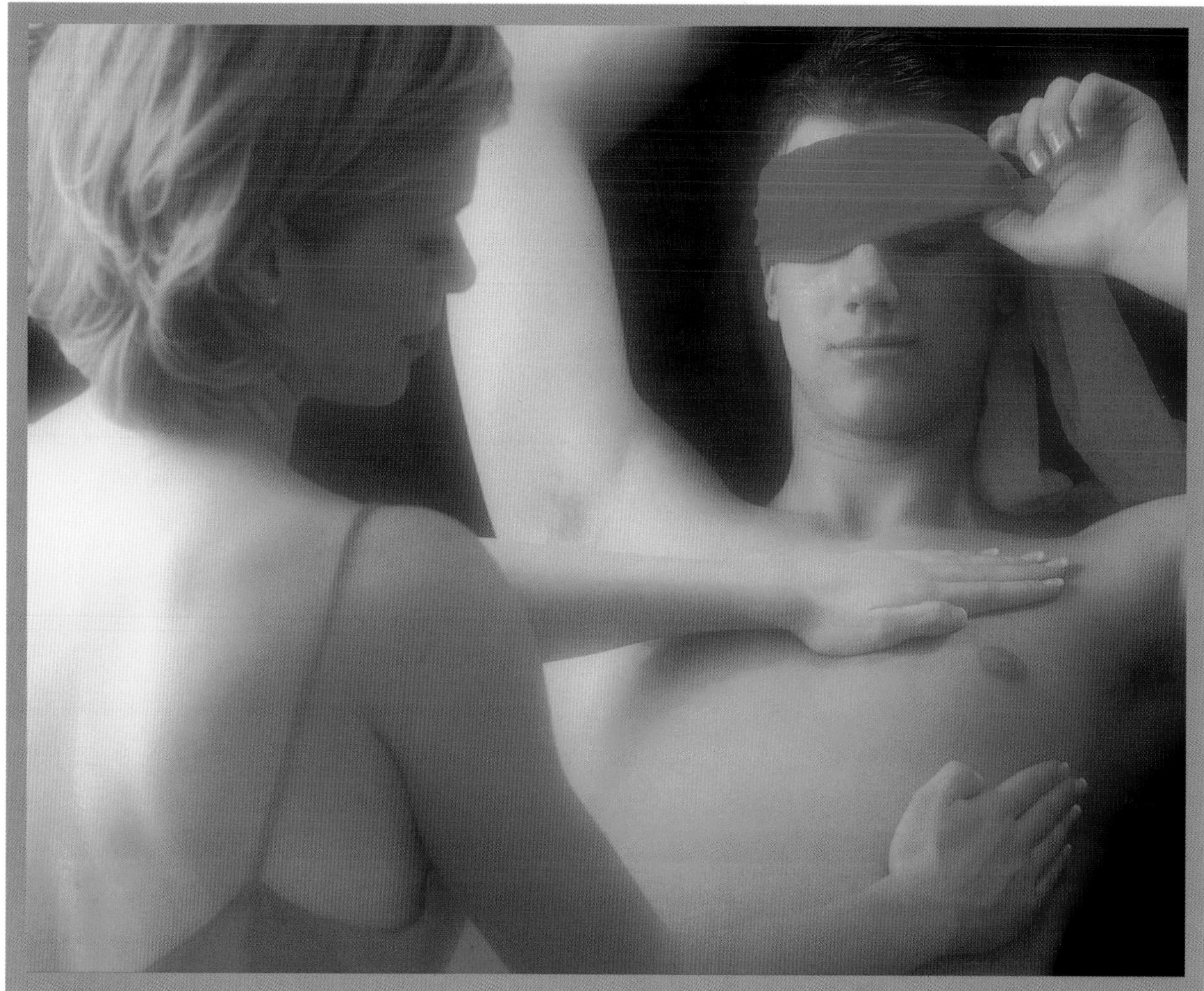

2 You are ready to begin focusing on just one side of the chest. Instead of gliding both hands in the same direction as before, place one hand more toward your lover's side and the other in the center of the chest. As you resume your effleurage stroke, the hand in the middle continues this long flowing motion between the nipples and up the arm closest to you. Your other hand travels the path of your original return stroke, down the arm over the armpit and along the side. As one hand travels up the chest and arm, the other travels down the arm and along the side. The return stroke is the same only in reverse down the arm and center of the chest while the other hand travels up along the side over the armpit and up the arm. These strokes are slow and deliberate, but because there is no feathering return stroke, the massage takes on a more concentrated and thorough feeling. This is your opportunity to help relax tension both in the chest muscles where they come off the breast bone, to the shoulder joint just beneath the collar bone, and in those same muscles from the side of the chest.

2a To vary this stroke, with each successive stroke inch your hands closer to breast tissue. First move the hand on the breast bone closer to the nipples and begin massaging directly over the chest (pectoralis major) muscles. The other hand along the side begins to scoop underneath the breast tissue during the course of its stroke. Both hands approach the breast simultaneously and almost lift the breast from its foundation, allowing the attachments of the breast to be relaxed fully. Remember that this stroke needs to be slow and deliberate. In this way, if your lover experiences any discomfort, the stroke can be halted.

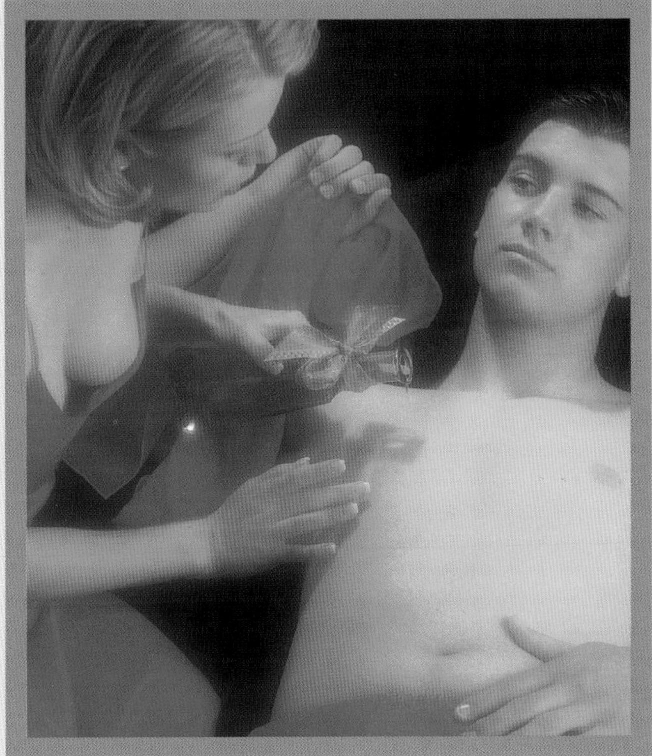

These next massage strokes are geared specifically to arouse erotic sensations in your lover. The nipples are highly sensitive in both men and women, so, just because this stroke involves the breast, do not exclude it from your male partner.

3 Make slow, feathering circles with your fingertips commencing at the outer edges of breast outlining tissue. Continue making the circles, smaller and smaller, slower and slower, until you reach the nipple. With each repeat of this stroke get closer to the nipple; first brush it, then touch it, finally drag over it.

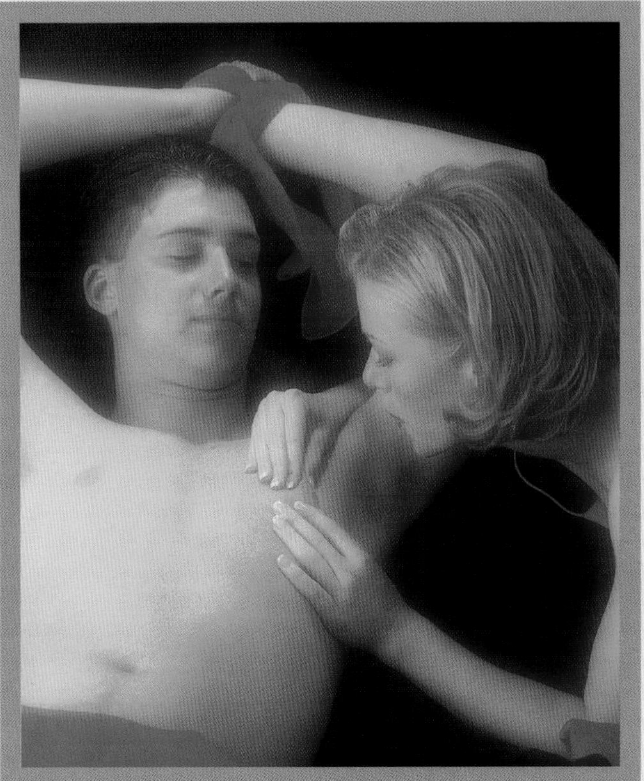

3a Now make "spoke strokes" on the nipple. With thumb and opposing fingers of each hand, lightly grasp the nipple and gently traction out away from its center; pull in opposite directions. Move a little, as if following the spokes of a bicycle and continue the stroke on each of the "spokes."

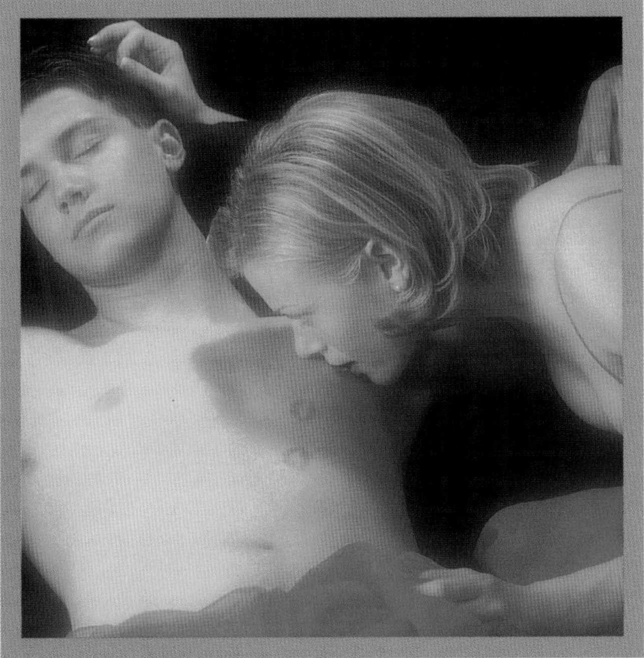

3b Finally, lightly grasp the nipple itself and ever so delicately traction the nipple up; lift it anywhere from a quarter to half an inch. Then let it go. If the release is abrupt or feels like snapping, you tractioned a little too much. You may use your thumb and finger or lips to traction the nipple. The nipples are very sensitive areas, and in foreplay and love making, these parts of the body can truly heighten the passion you both feel. Repeat the chest sequence on the other side.

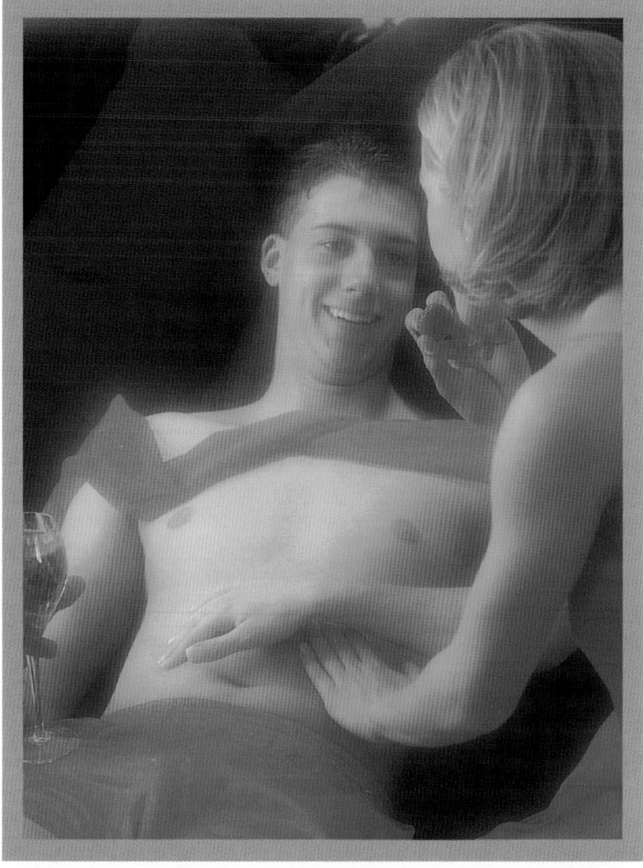

The abdomen is as sensitive and vulnerable as the chest. It is our seat of power, speaking emotionally. We hold our insecurities, our fears, our worries, and our anxieties in this area. We are apprehensive about people touching us there. We become ticklish as a protective response. You should approach the abdomen with great respect and reverence, because your lover is allowing you into their personal, most private of spaces to enjoy and express warm feelings of love. Touching them with any other regard, no matter what the intention, can violate trust in you as a partner and affect your relationship.

4 Apply oil, with your hands to the abdomen in a circular motion. The circle should be clockwise, because the digestive process of the intestines and bowels moves clockwise. Counterclockwise might cause discomfort if food is present. Move the hands in a "sun and moon" pattern one hand creates a full circle on the abdomen; the other hand half circles as the first hand completes the second half of its initial revolution. Repeat this for several minutes. It is very soothing and allows your lover to trust your touch there.

5 Now make small circles in a circular pattern around the navel. Four to six inches out from the navel, press points, and make circles on the points in a circle. This can soothe cramps and digestive pains.

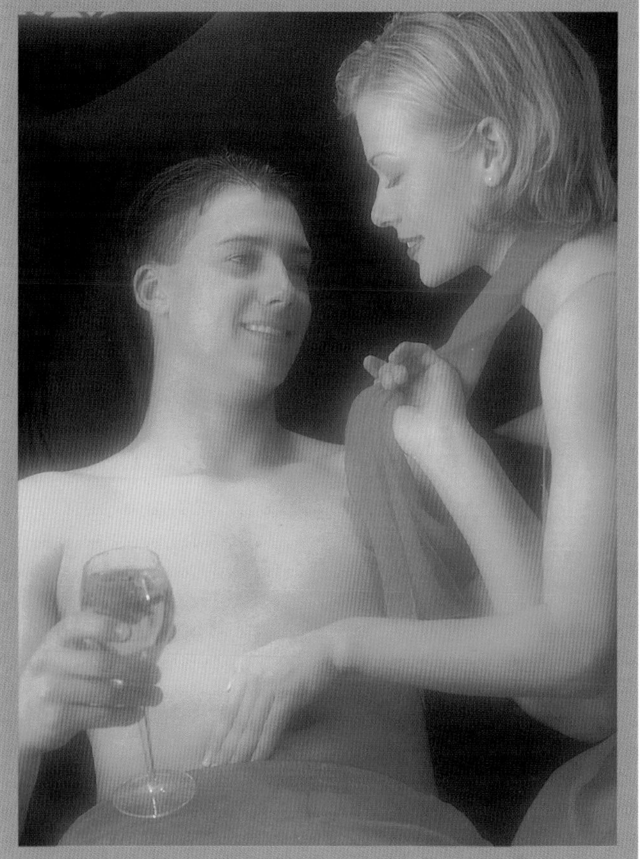

Do you have a "Minimum Daily Requirement of Romance?"

- *What is your partner's "Minimum Daily Requirement of Romance?'*
- *How does your weekly, monthly, or yearly need of romance compare with your partner's need?*
- *Take the time to discuss where the balance is so that romantic needs are being met.*
- *Plan ahead for some of your romantic interludes, and allow others to happen spontaneously.*

6 Now milk the sides of your partner. This is done by reaching over them to their opposite side with one hand, tucking your fingers slightly under them and pulling back in a smooth effleurage stroke. As your first hand reaches midway across their body, begin the same stroke with the other hand, always pulling toward you. Start just above the hip bone and continue upward to the chest and back down again.

6a A variation of this milking stroke is called raking, which is performed the same way, but with fingers spread apart and firmer pressure. As you approach the rib cage, your fingers seem to fit between each of the ribs. Moving too quickly with this stroke can be ticklish, so use slow and deliberate strokes up the sides from just above the hip to the chest and back again. Remember to do this stroke and the milking stroke on both sides of the body.

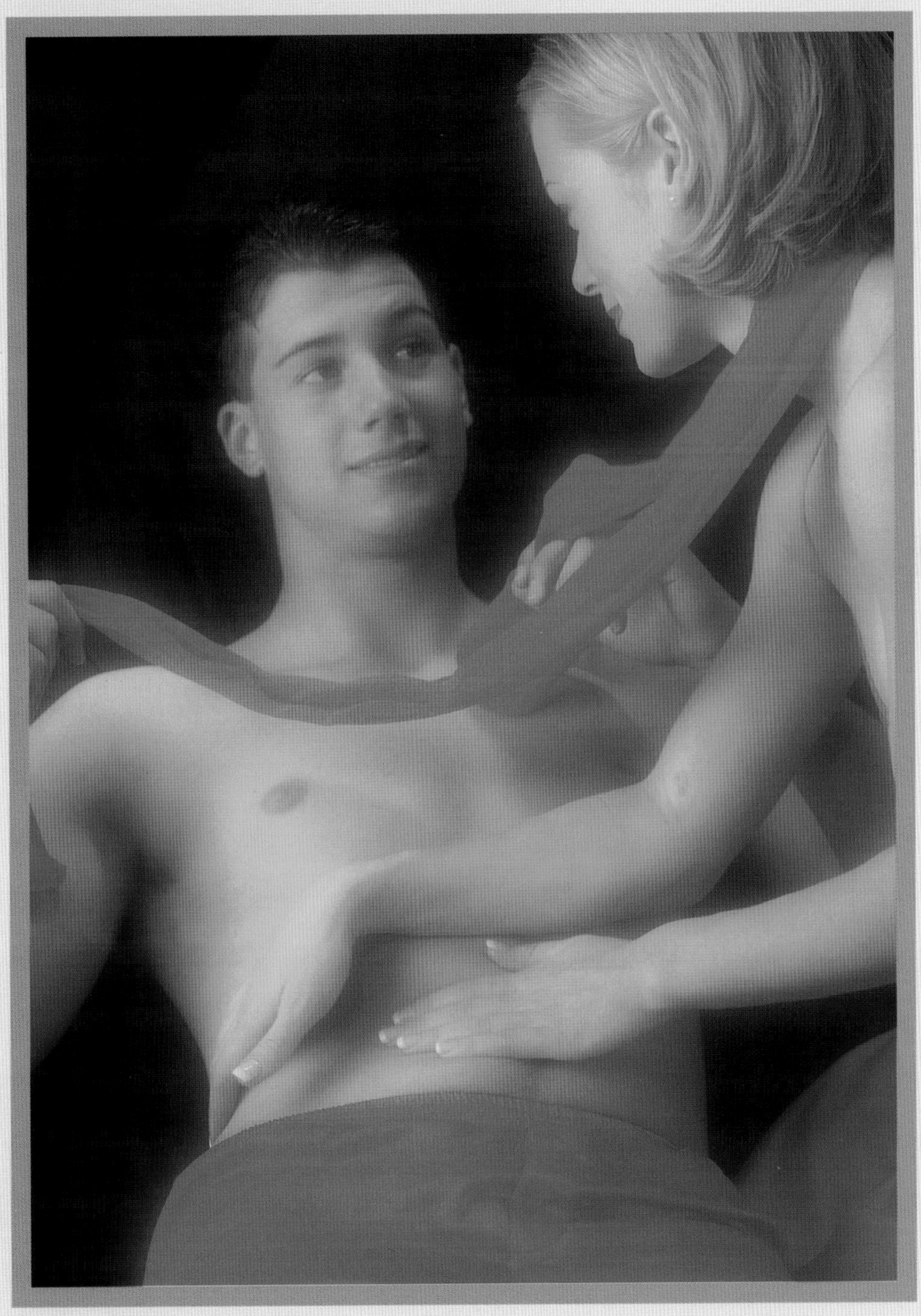

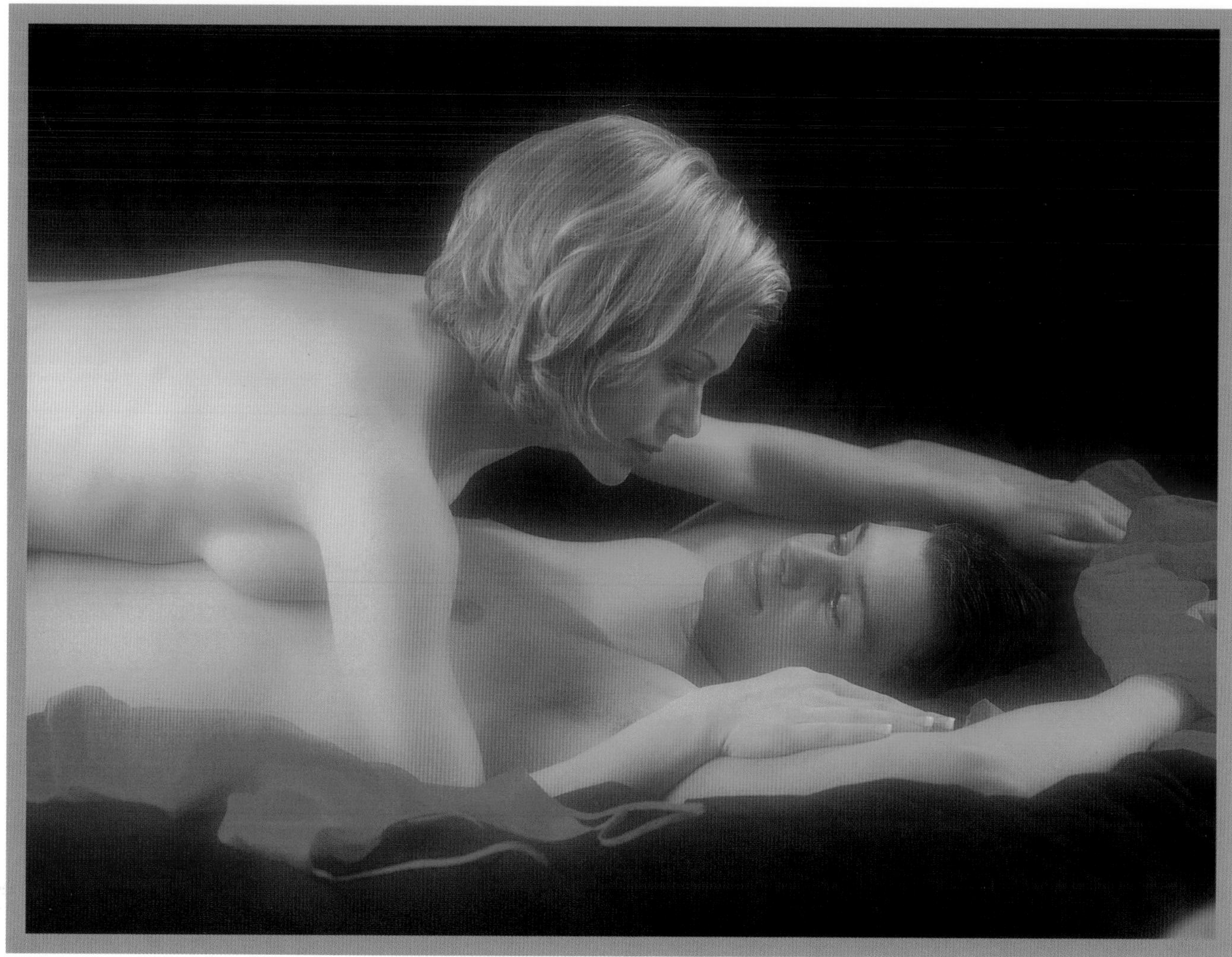

7 As the massage of your lover's front side is almost complete and their arms are extended over their head and to their sides, you may perform a full-body effleurage stroke from head to toe. First start with your hands on both ankles. Begin to glide your hands up their legs, along the folds dividing their thighs and abdomen. Bringing your hands together, continue the stroke up their tummy between their breasts, and out and up their arms as far as you can comfortably reach. Return with light feathering down the arms, over the armpit, along the sides, down the abdomen, toward the groin, along the inner thighs and along the legs to the tips of the toes.

With each successive stroke, glide slower and lighter, both on the up stroke and the return. Create subtle variations where your hands brush up against your lover's genitals, nipples, armpits, neck, and ears. Move lighter and slower each time until you feel like movement is imperceptible. You can perform this stroke ten times or more.

Full Moon Bath

2 cups sea salt　6 drops wintergreen oil　6 drops bayberry oil　6 drops amergris oil　6 drops sage oil

As the full moon rises, you may want to try a Full Moon Bath. While running the bath, add sea salt and essential oils. Gently swirl bath until oils and salt is dissolved. Light a tall white candle and dim the lights. Other mood enhancers could be background flute music and a warm cup of soothing tea such as chamomile.

8 Another full-body stroke requires you to be positioned at your lover's head. Lubricate your hands and arms up to the elbow. With their arms still extended, reach as far down their body as possible, usually to about the hips, and place your hands under the buttocks at the gluteal crack on either side. With your hands facing palm up, and curving your fingers only, lift at the finger and/or wrist joints, and begin to effleurage slowly up on either side of the spine. This gently stretches back muscles and tractions the spine to allow nerves to breathe easier. Continue the stroke up toward the shoulder blade, and then glide your hands apart and out to the sides of their body. You may even continue the stroke up the arms and connect with their hands for a moment or two. Do this once, maybe twice.

8a While at their head, reach down the spine on either side between their shoulder blades. You may only be able to reach as far as midback to just above the buttocks. Again, curve your fingers and lift only with your fingers or wrist joints. Begin tractioning up the back. This will make your lover's back arch and tip their chin up. Move slowly and in a flowing manner. This variation of the previous body stretch feels great, as if one is being suspended and floating. You will notice your face is very close to their chest and mouth during this stroke. Take advantage of the moment and arouse your lover with hot passionate breaths, gentle kisses, teasing nibbles, and tantalizing licks.

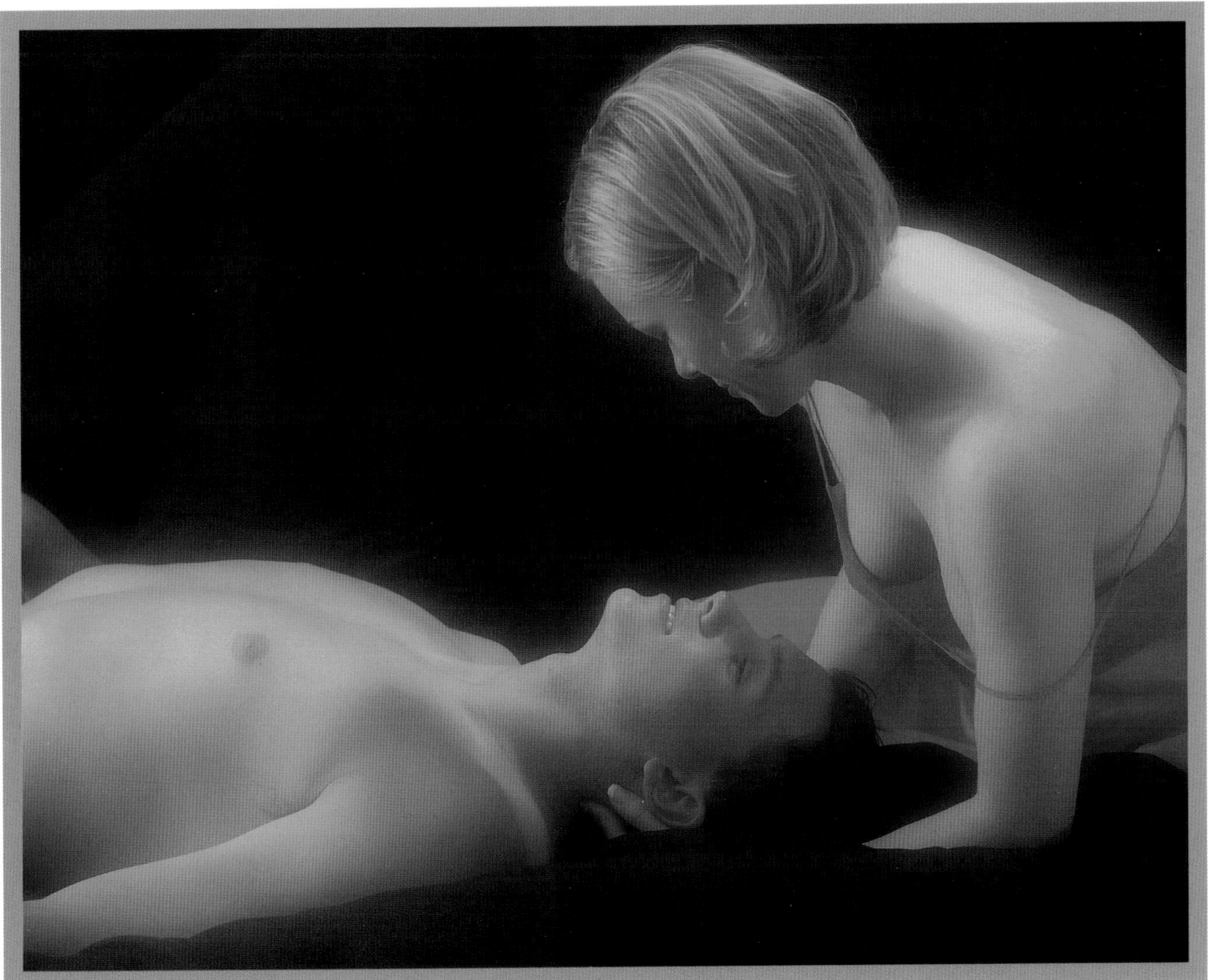

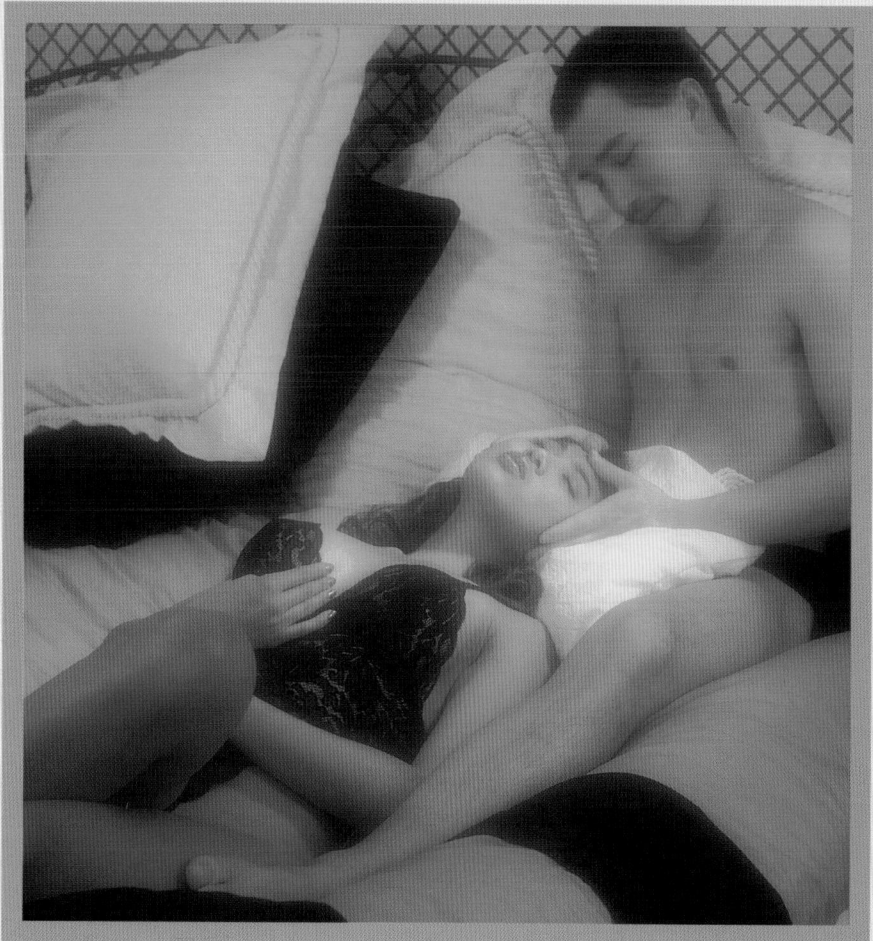

Face & Scalp

No massage is complete without addressing the face and scalp. In fact, you can make an entire massage out of doing the neck and shoulders followed by the face and scalp. It is a fabulous massage session to ease headache pain and muscle tension from stress. Just like a foot bath and massage, the neck and shoulder sequence followed by the face and scalp is very relaxing after a hard day at work.

1 At your lover's head, without using any oil, lay your thumbs flat on the center of the forehead. Use flowing strokes to draw the thumbs out toward the temples. Imagine you are ironing out the stress and tension of the day as you repeat this stroke.

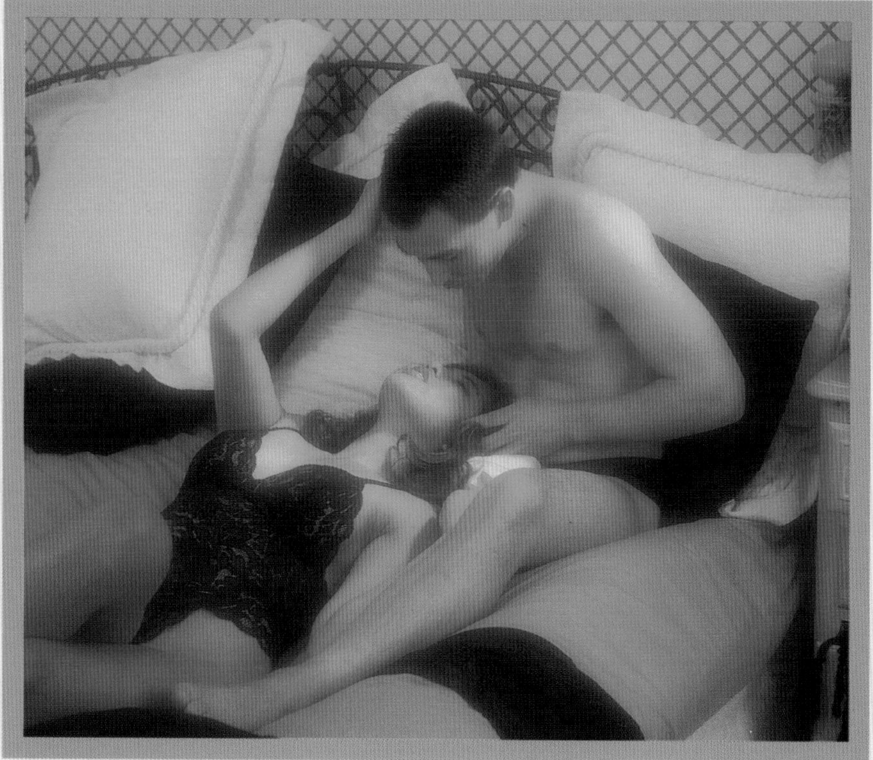

2 On your last stroke on the forehead, move your index, middle, and ring fingers together directly over your lover's temples on either side of their head. Make medium-size circles around their temples very slowly — the slower, the better. You can repeat this for several minutes. you can change the direction of the circles by having both hands move together, then alternating one clockwise and the other counterclockwise, and back and forth again. This stroke has a mesmerizing affect on people. It melts tension headaches away quite easily.

3 Now, smooth the nose and cheeks. Using the same technique on the nose as you did on the forehead, glide gently down your lover's face on either side of their nose. Before you get to the nostrils, rotate your thumbs; lay them flat on the cheekbones, and smooth out the skin along the face down to and including the jawbone. Repeat this stroke several times. You may play with their lips as you outline them in a feathering technique and gently pull them apart.

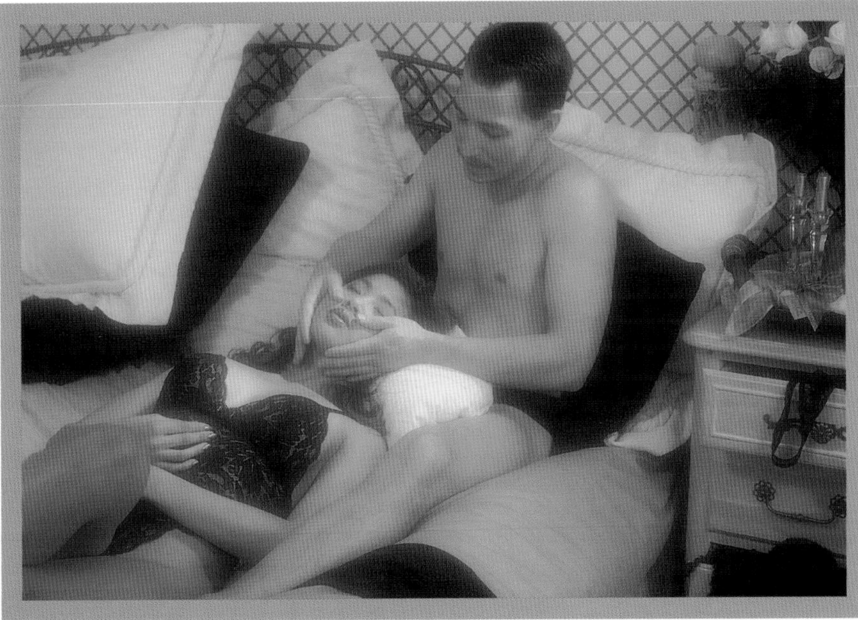

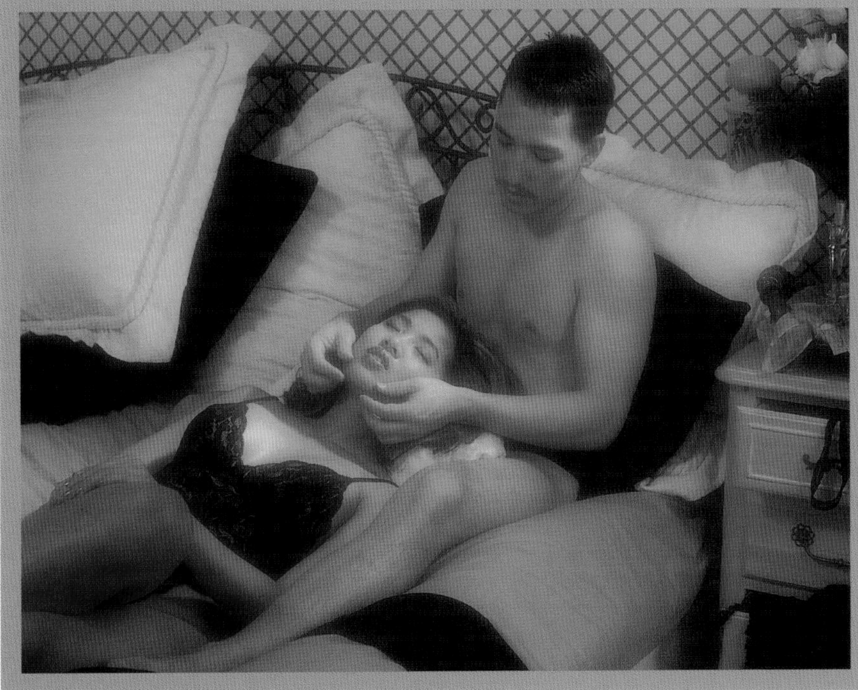

4 Bring your thumb, index, and middle fingers together to form what is called "kitty paws." Gently squeeze your lover's chin between the kitty paws using both your hands on either side of the chin. Continue this kitty paw squeeze technique along their chin and up the jaw to where the jawbone hinges, below their temples. The thumb should be on top of the chin and the finger below the chin bone. Now follow the bone up and around to just beneath the ear. You can even tease and tickle their ears after doing kitty paws several times.

A Few Romantic Suggestions:

- *Watching a sunrise or sunset*
- *A soft touch*
- *A "certain" look*
- *Any kind of flowers*
- *Taking a walk together*
- *Breakfast in bed*
- *Love notes or love letters*
- *Candlelight dinner*
- *Picnic for two*
- *Surprise tickets to an exotic place*
- *Phone call just to say "I love you."*
- *Home alone—just the two of you*
- *Glass of wine to share*
- *Music (your romantic taste)*
- *Moonlight walks*
- *The smell of cologne or perfume*
- *Bubblebaths*
- *Carriage rides*
- *Dancing*
- *Old romantic movies*
- *Whipped cream and strawberries*
- *"Pet" names*
- *Cuddling*
- *Chocolate*

5 Place your hands on either side of the base of your partner's head, and tip their head to one side as you catch it with your other hand. With your one hand cradling the head, you will notice the neck is now exposed. Take a small amount of oil to lubricate your free hand and, using the thumb and opposing fingers stroke the neck downward with long flowing glides. Do not press too deeply with your thumb; it might restrict your partner's airway slightly. Repeat this stroke several times.

6 Reverse the neck stroke from a downward pattern to an upward stroke. Pressure is deeper as the hand and finger lift the neck and shoulder muscles from the shoulder joint toward the base of the neck and up to the base of the skull. This stroke feels absolutely luxurious. You may repeat this as many times as you or your partner would like.

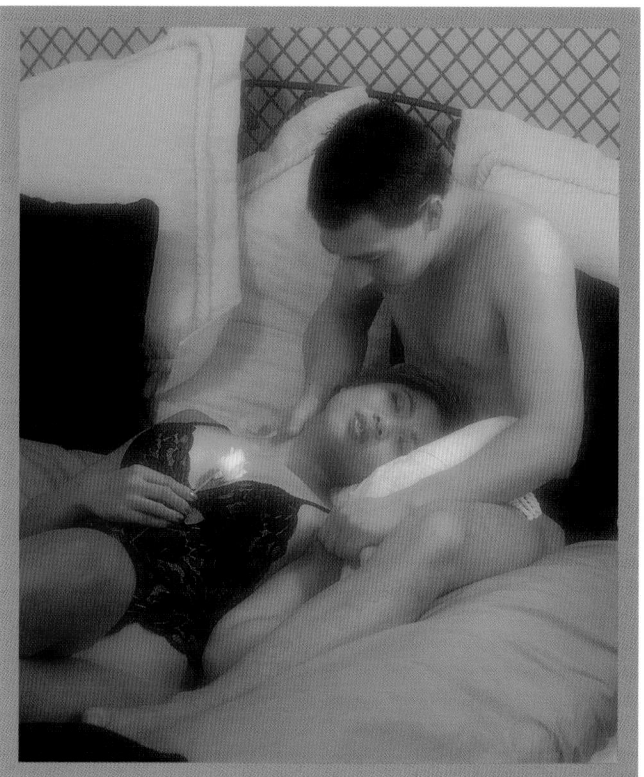

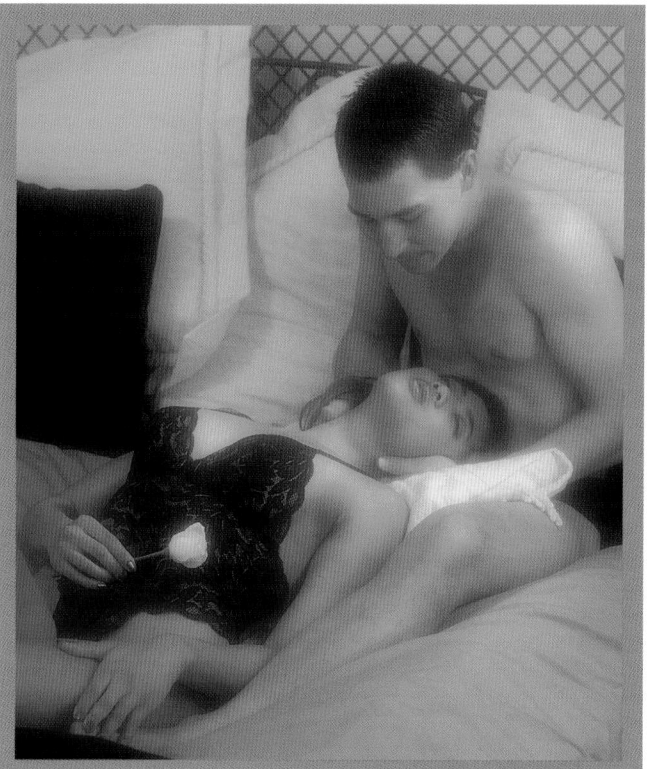

Set the mood with one or more of these albums:

Amore: The Great Italian Love Arias	*Reflections of Passion, Yanni*
Feels So Good, Chuck Mangione	*Something of Time, Nightnoise*
Livin' Inside your Love, George Benson	*Optimystique, Yanni*
Autumn, George Winston	*Kiss Under the Moon, Warren Hill*
The Pachelbel Canon, Johann Pachelbel	*Unforgettable, Natalie Cole*
Power of Love, Luther VanDross	*Heartsounds, David Lanz*
Time, Lives, and Tenderness, Michael Bolton	*Your favorite romantic movie sound track*

7 While the base of your partner's skull is exposed during the neck stroke, use your fingers to make circular motions along the muscles that attach to the back of the skull. These muscles get quite tense when someone becomes stressed. The tight muscles will, over time, produce a headache that travels forward from the back of the head over the scalp to the front of the head. Press firmly as you use circular friction from behind the ear to the center of the back of the head. You may hear groans of delight as these muscles begin to release their tension and the blood begins to flow easier.

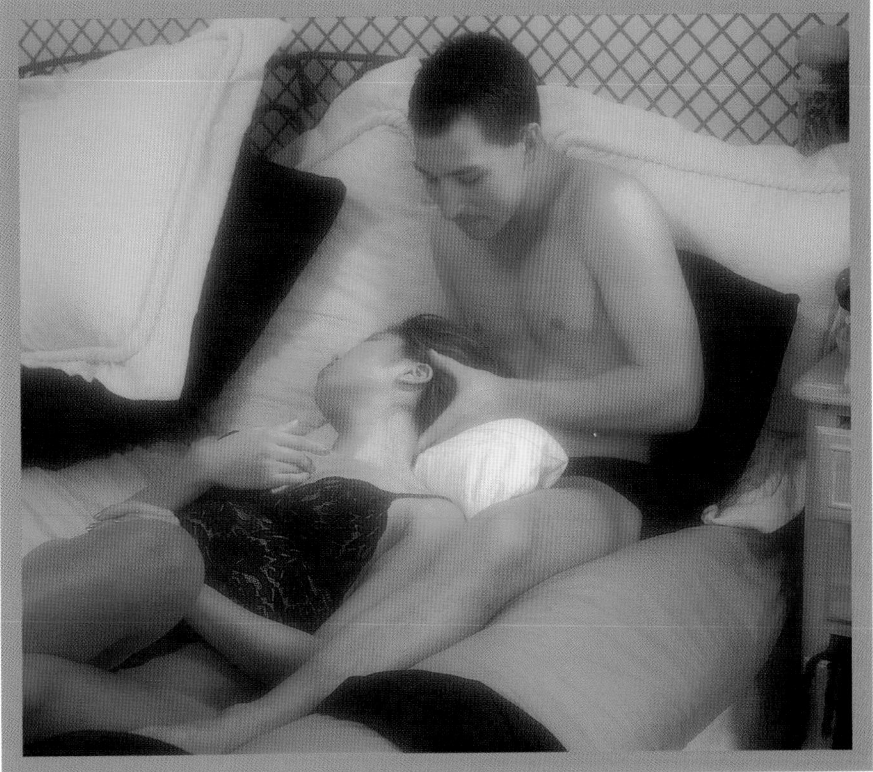

8 The last stroke of our romantic massage focuses on the scalp. Place your fingers on the scalp and massage gently as if you were shampooing the hair, only more slowly. It is so soothing to have someone stroke your head like this; it can easily mesmerize your lover. Massage the entire scalp from the base of the skull up and over the sides of the head and to the forehead. Even if your lover has receding hair, massage the skin of the scalp. It feels so good! When you are finished, do not forget to turn their head to the other side for face and scalp sequence.

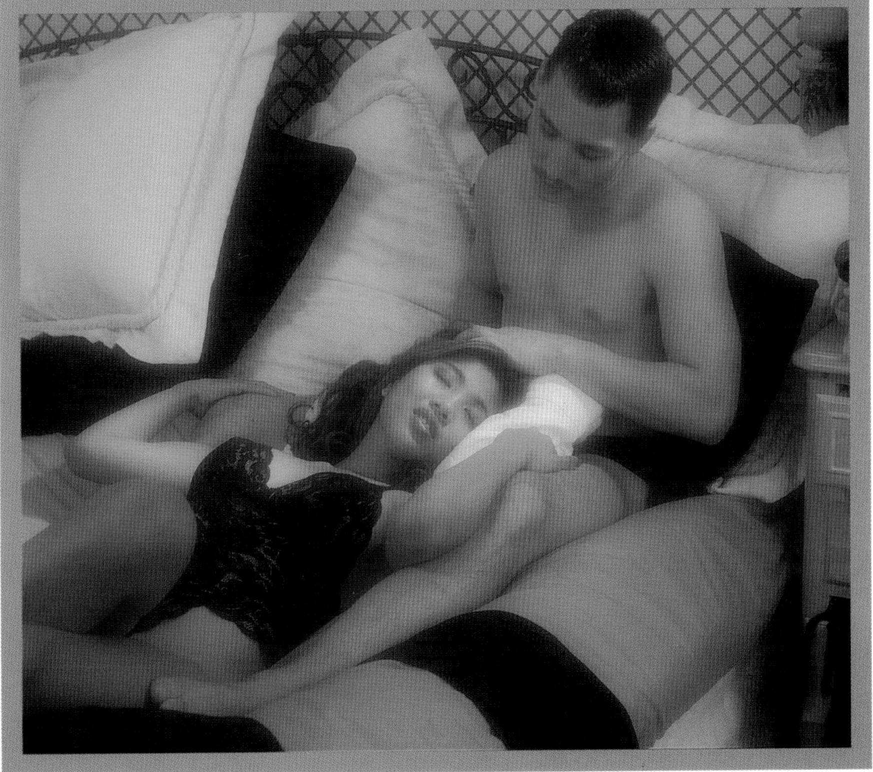

A good relationship allows both partners to "be themselves" without the need or desire for pretenses. A "true love" allows you to let your guard down and say what is on your mind.

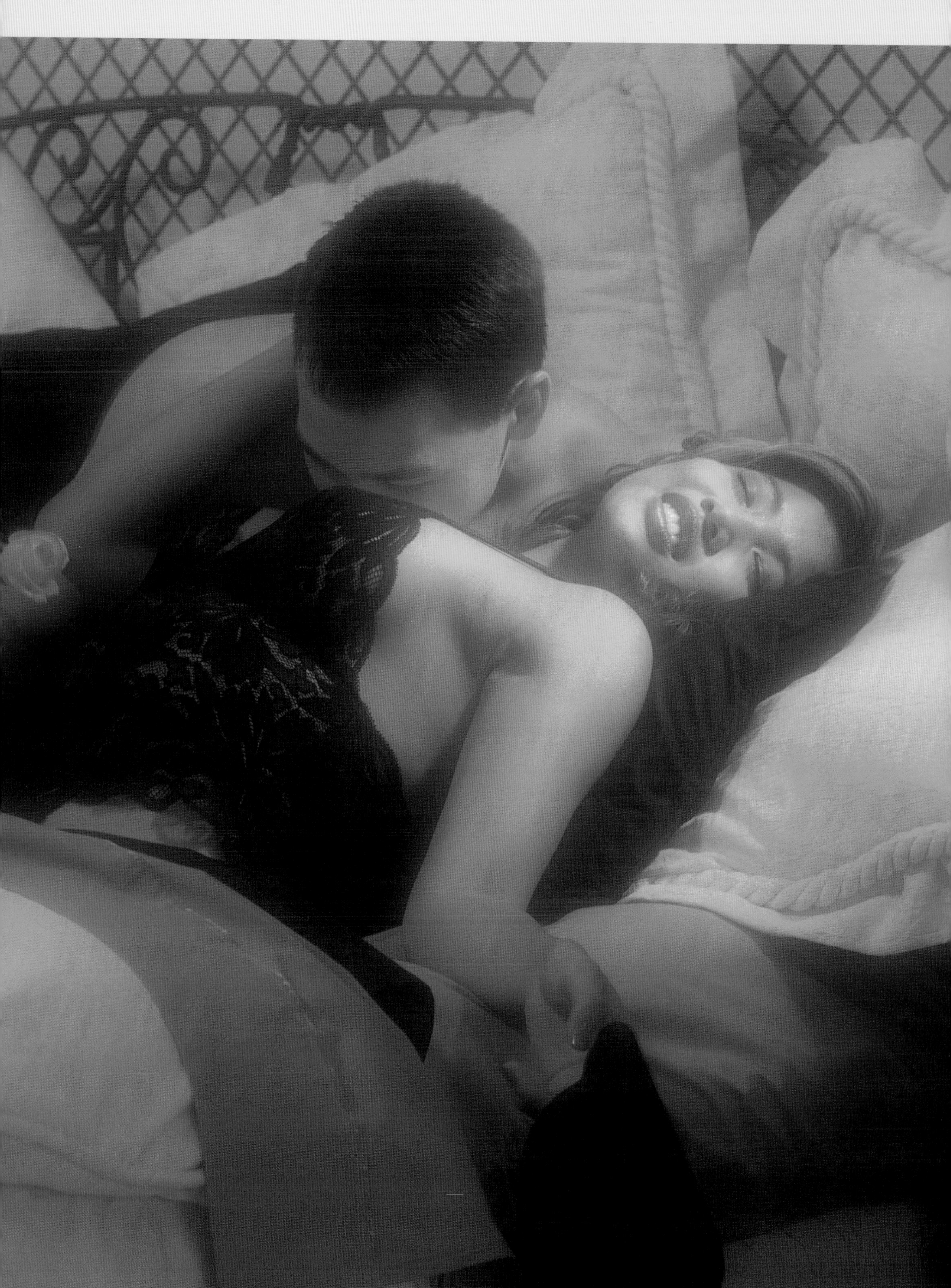

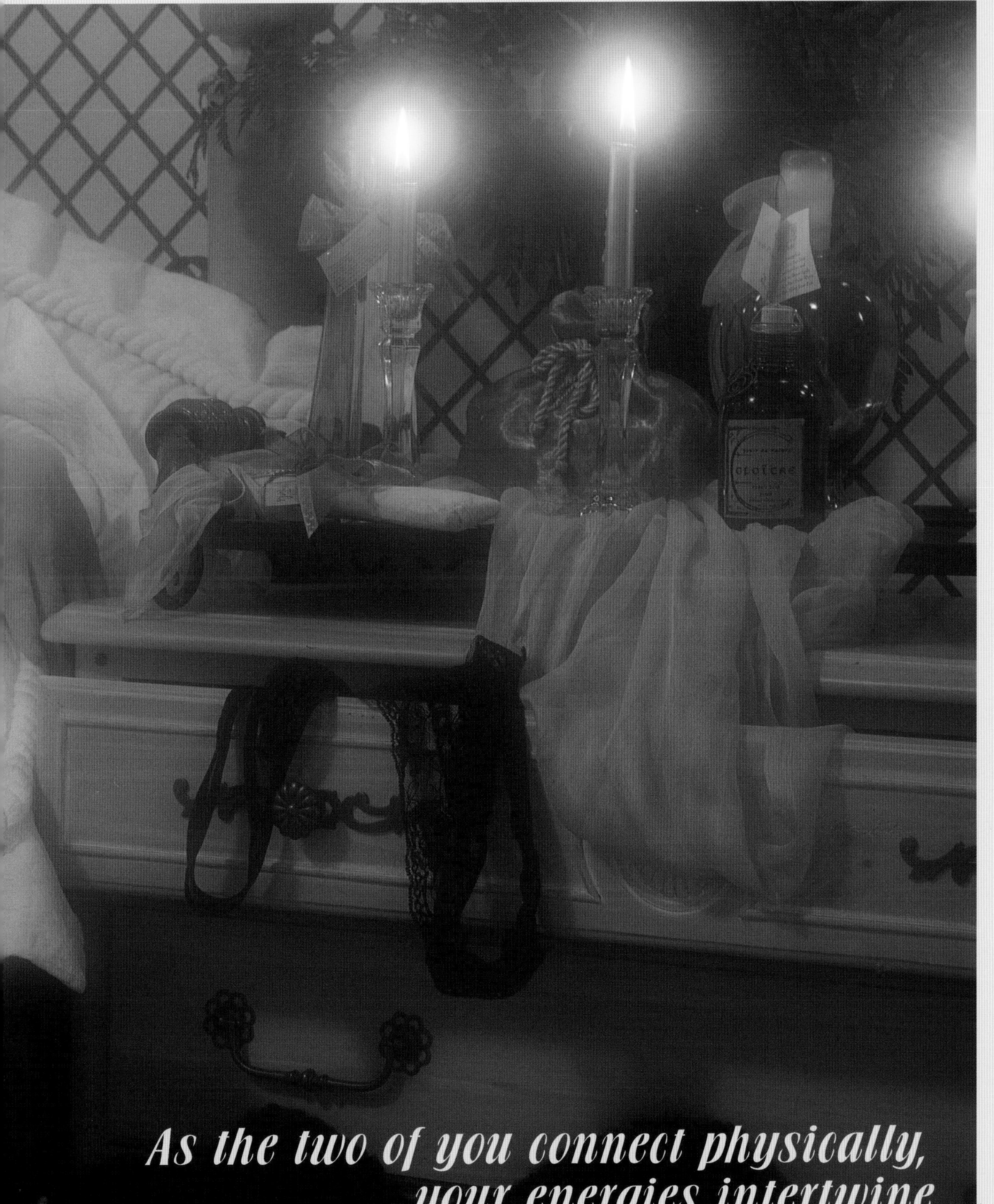

*As the two of you connect physically,
your energies intertwine
in united love.*

chapter eight

Connecting Holds

As your romantic massage comes to a conclusion, there are certain sensitive connecting holds that will help relax, as well as unite, the two of you. These connecting holds involve bio-electric energy fields that interweave as you become closer and establish a connection with one another.

Your body's bio-energy field, or aura, has several centers of electric emittance. The Hindus call these centers, chakras and they include:

- ♥ **Crown** of the head connects you to all that is spiritual
- ♥ **Third eye** represents intuition (located between the eye brows, approximately 1" above the bridge of nose)
- ♥ **Throat** allows one to communicate freely either in speech or written communication
- ♥ **Heart center** emanates love, compassion, and nurturing
- ♥ **Solar plexus** connects to happiness and joy, the true source of power (located in the abdomen)

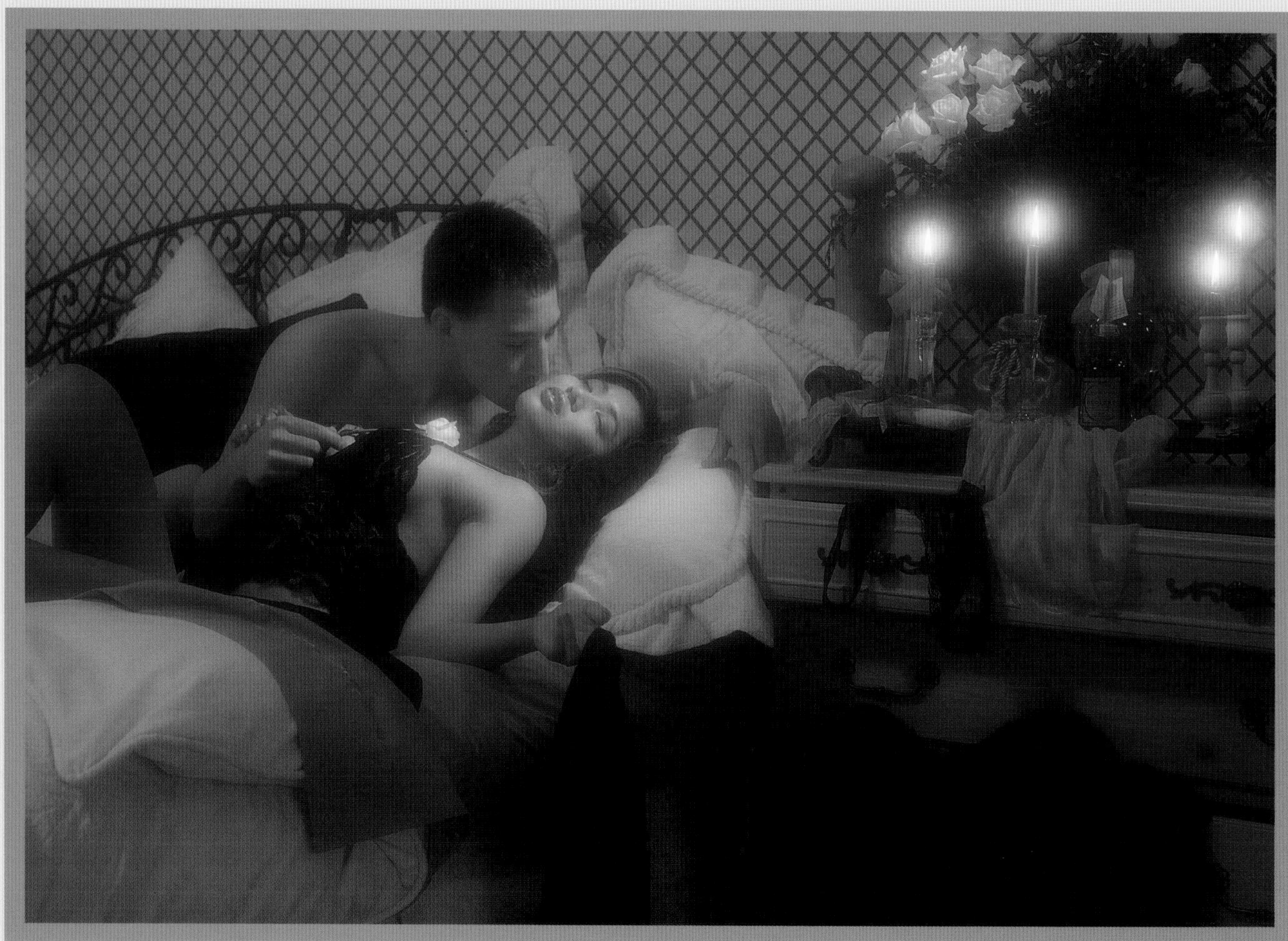

- ♥ **Hara** (Chinese derivative) is where our life force and sexual energy originate
- ♥ **Root** connects us to the earth and keeps us grounded and stable.

By connecting with these energy centers, these chakras, on our lover, we can affect them as we affect ourselves. This can sound a bit mystical, but has existed in traditional Chinese medicine for over 5,000 years, and has been documented throughout the world. We understand that there are many forces of natural science and physics that are not visible; auras exist and have been proven scientifically in the medical profession. Therapeutic Touch, which is practiced in many hospitals, affects the auras, which in turn affects a patients' health.

The holds described in this chapter will have varying effects on your partner and yourself. Be sensitive to any feelings, impressions, or sensations you both may experience.

Holding the Crown

At your partner's head, place both of your thumbs at the very apex of the head. This is located by finding the top most part of the ears on either side, and tracing a line up over the head simultaneously. Where your fingers meet is the crown of the head. This massage is very calming and enhances one's spirituality. If you are sensitive and have a sense of intuition, you may connect with your lover, begin feeling their emotions, or pick up on their thoughts.

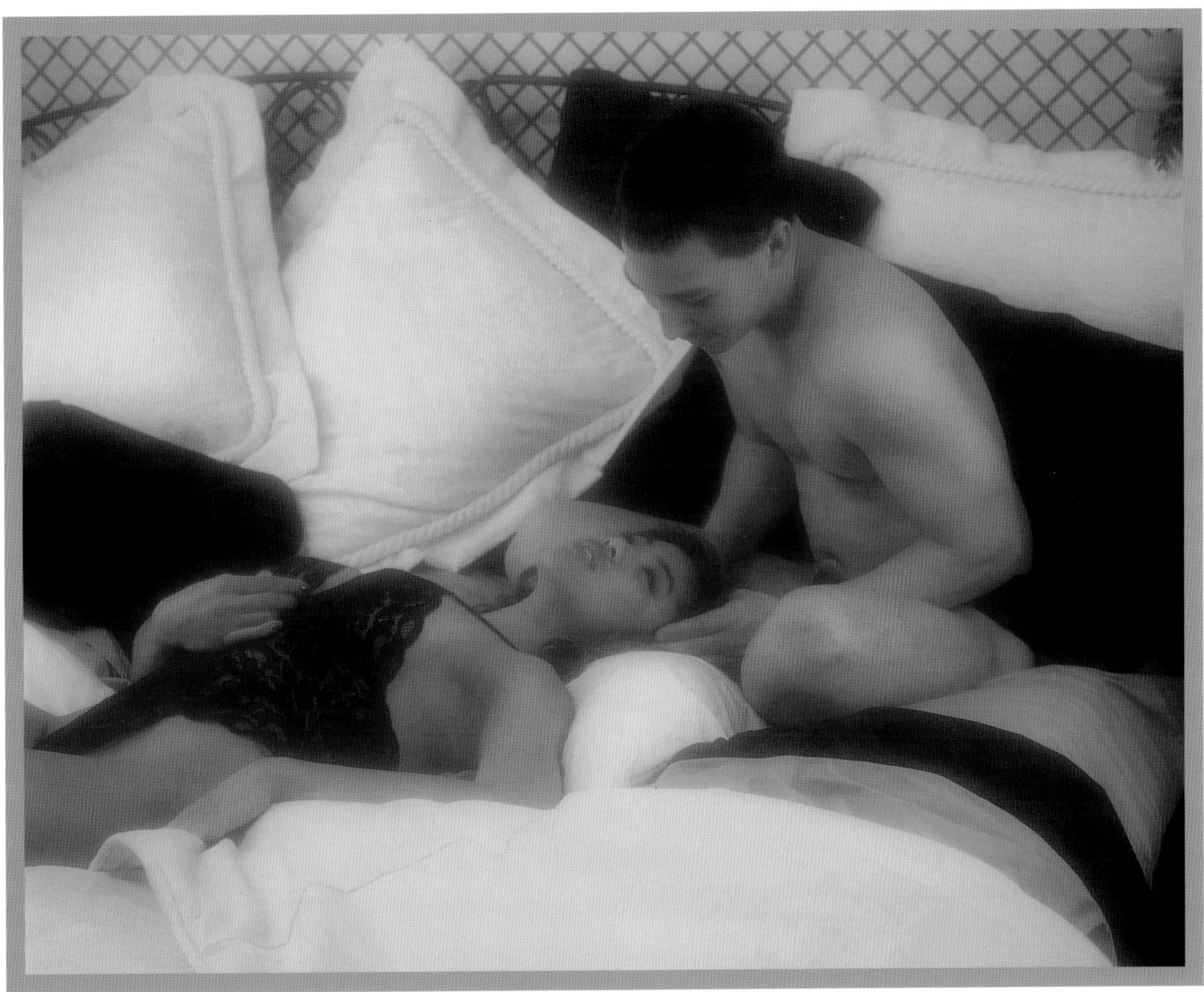

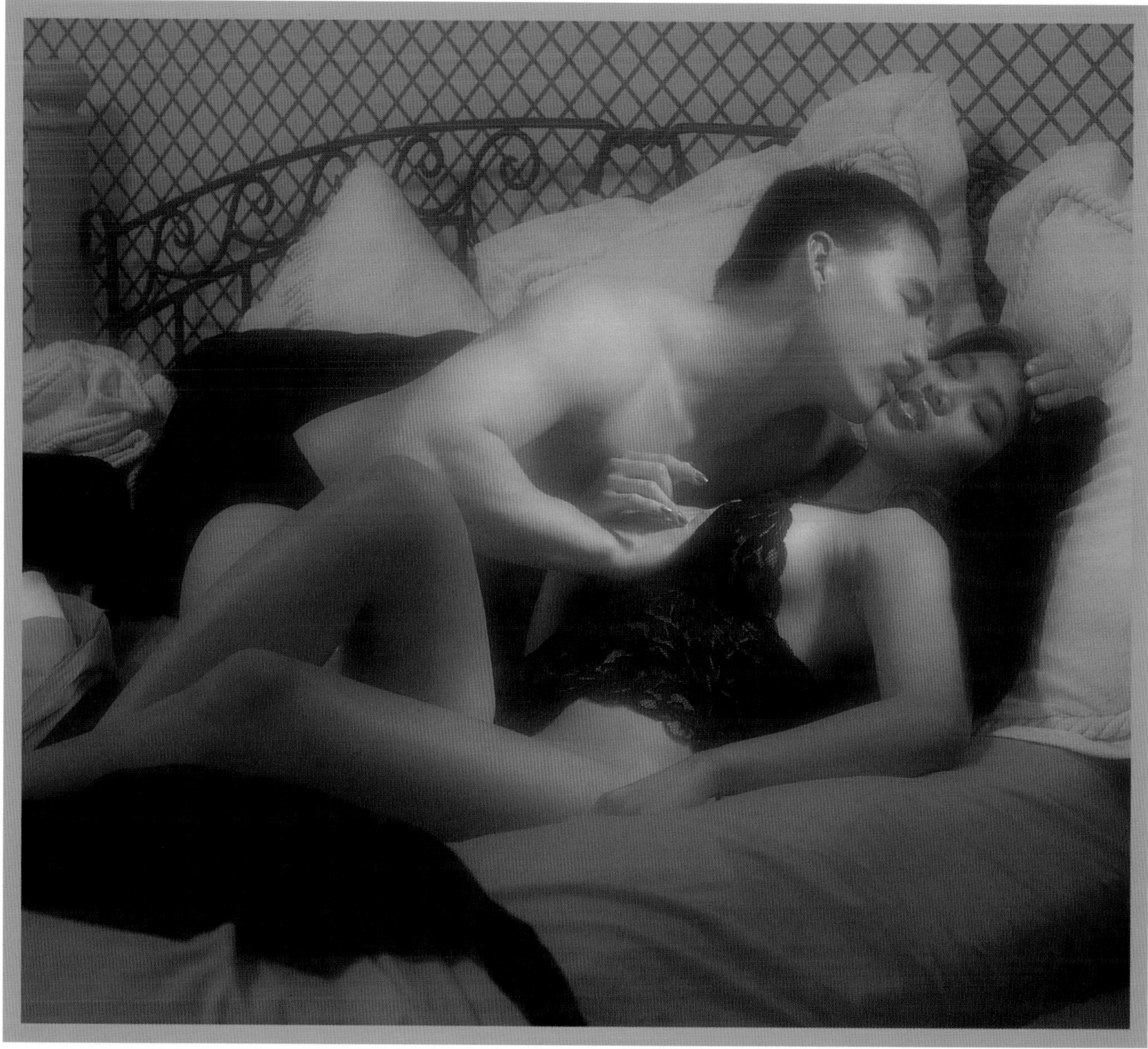

Crown & Heart

Holding the crown of your lover's head with your left hand and placing your right hand on the center of their chest between the nipples activates inner peace and tranquility.

These two energy centers — the crown and heart — are well known in acupuncture and acupressure which use thumb or finger pressure to activate oriental acupoints to promote health and well-being. They are used in Chinese medicine to calm the heart and mind. These are the most calming points on the body. These two points held together can relax someone who has been traumatized, or who is experiencing anxiety or nervousness.

Using the crown and heart center hold on your lover allows them to relax, and reach a profound level of peace and security as you nurture those needs in them. Hold the points for several minutes. You may feel a warmth in your hands resembling your partner's body heat. You may also notice a tingly, electric, buzzy feeling; or a pulsing that does not normally follow their heart beat.

Crown, Third Eye, Throat, & Heart

This next hold connects all of the higher chakras in peaceful, loving moods, while allowing your partner's intuition to speak freely to their mind.

With your left hand, use the thumb to hold the crown and middle finger to hold the third eye point. Now, with your right hand, place your thumb at the notch between the collar bones while the middle finger connects with the heart center. This hold can be maintained for five minutes or more.

While connecting with your partner in this way, they are able to reach a deep meditative state. They can become aligned to a higher sense of self, a vision of truth, a stability of self worth and love, and an openness to understanding and communication. During this hold, you can connect to your lover in understanding their spirit, their perspective, their love — those things that they hold dear — and, of course, their expression of all these things to your mind, your inner self.

Use your breathing to move energy and feelings through your right hand to their heart. Allow this energy to rise within them as it connects with their thoughts and enters your left hand at their crown.

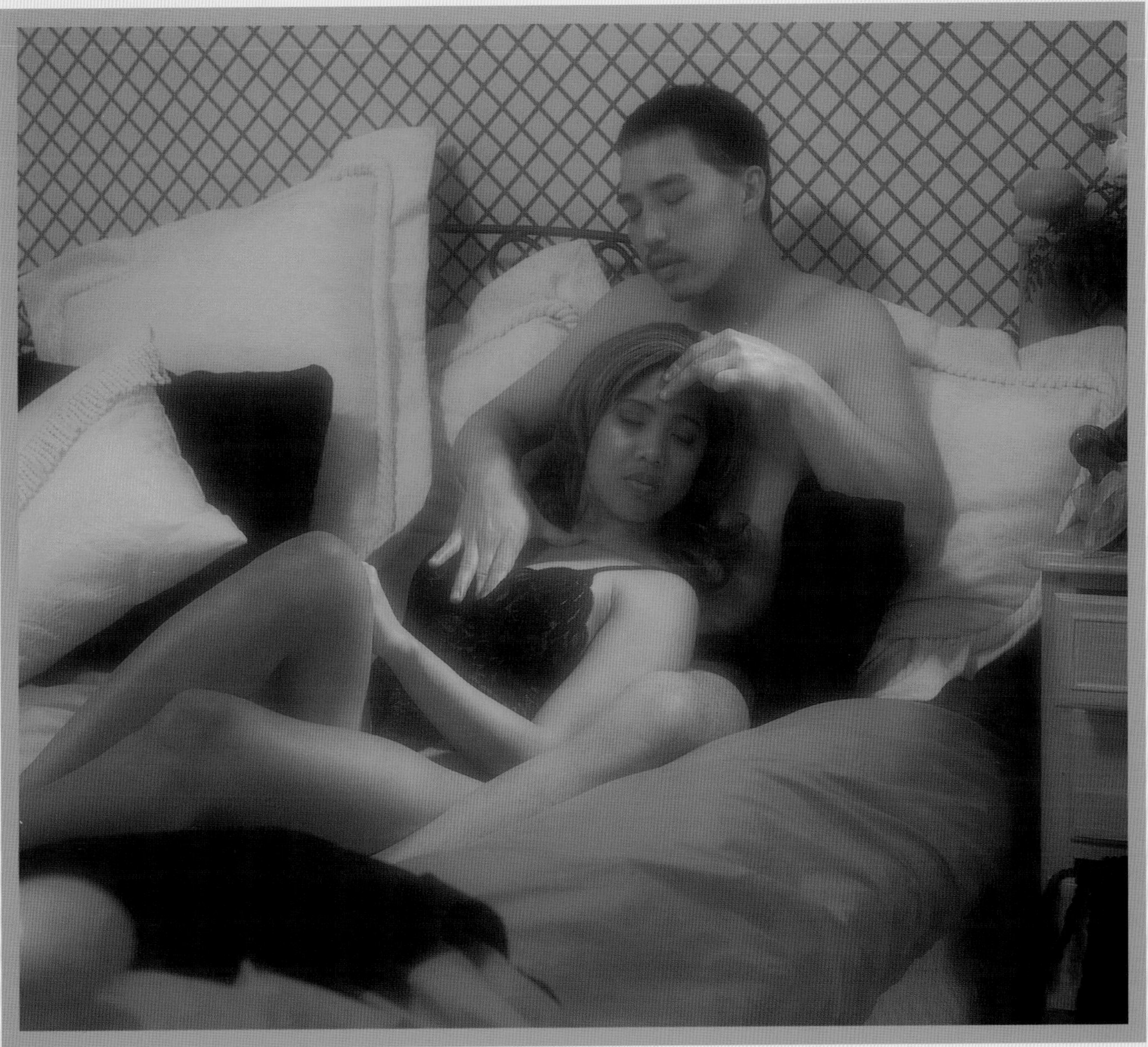

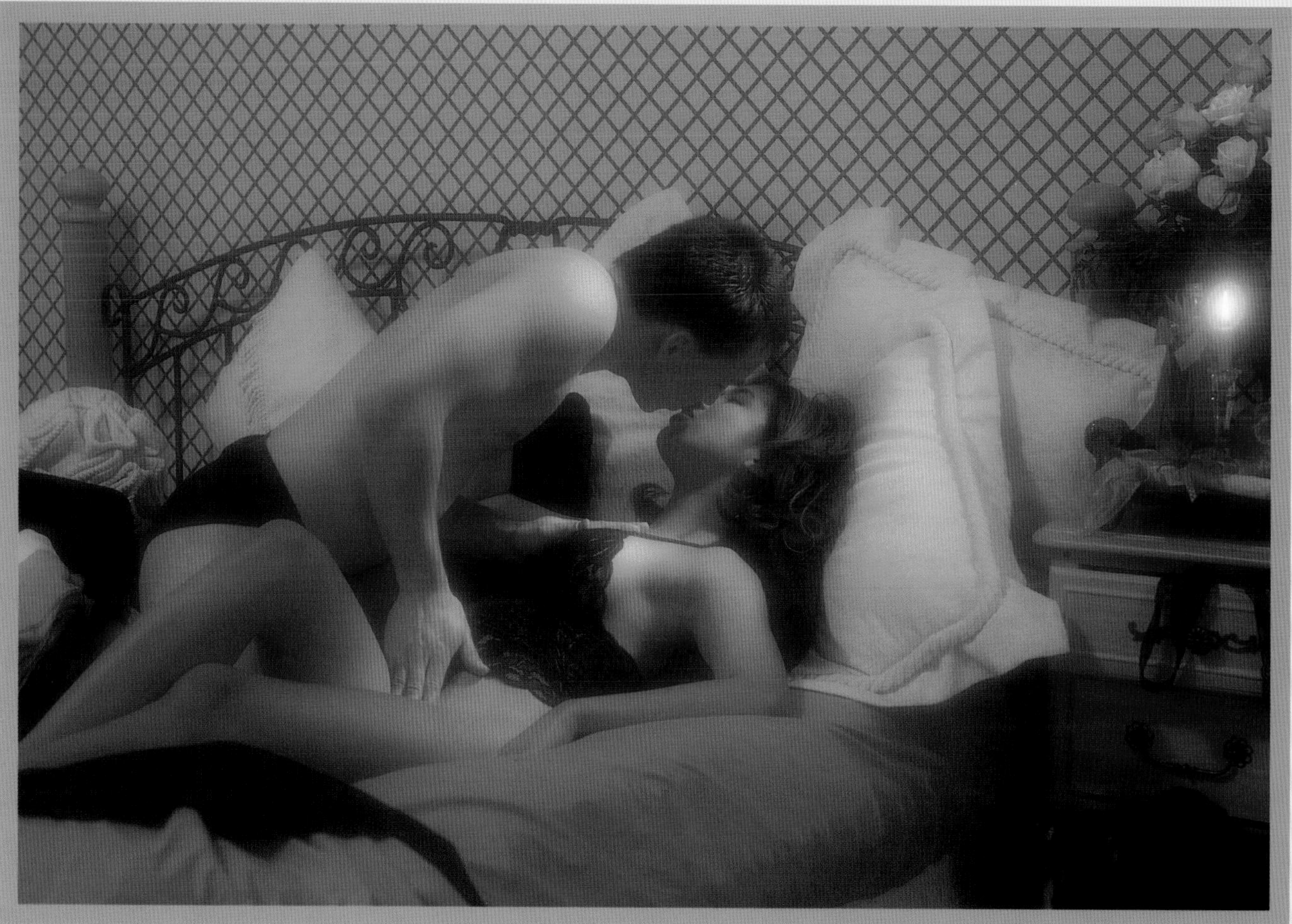

Heart Center & Root

This hold has its origins in the Tantric massage of India. Tantric practices use sexual union to reach a connection with the divine in all of us.

This erotic hold can stir sexual feelings in your lover, and should be used not as a calming hold after the massage, but during romantic massage to arouse their feelings of sexual desire and pleasure. Place your right hand on their genitals and your left hand over their heart center.

Align both of your breathing patterns out of sync, so that as you exhale your lover inhales. With every breath imagine energy moving. As you inhale, imagine energy from the world around you entering your body and metamorphosing into feelings of intimacy and sexual desire for your lover. With every exhalation, imagine sending this sexually stimulating energy out your right hand, into your lover's sex organs, and stirring something primitive and highly erotic within them. Also imagine that this Tantric energy rises in them to their heart center where it mingles with their loving emotions and feelings for you. That energy recirculates back to you through your left hand as you inhale, amplifies, and transmits back to them as you exhale and they inhale.

At this same time, your lover should be doing their own breathing and imagining. They should imagine this sexual energy flowing through your warm and loving hands into their genitals, stirring intimate feelings for you, rising within them to intensify feelings of love for you and sending it back to you through your left hand on their chest.

As you both enjoy this holding time, this breathing and sensual meditation, you may allow your hands to move and lightly massage in loving ways to help stimulate your partner's sexual excitation.

Crown & Root

This hold also has its origins in India, but is not a Tantric, or sexual hold. Even though the root chakra is accessed at the genitals, it does not necessarily stimulate sexual arousal. The root chakra is one of groundedness and stability. It represents the will to live, to manifest, to survive.

The crown chakra exemplifies spirituality, enlightenment, wisdom, and awareness of self truth. Holding both crown and root centers grounds their spirituality in the present. Your partner becomes more self-aware. The pleasures experienced in their body and their joy is complete in your expression of center. Instead of touching the genitals as in the last hold, place your right hand just above the genitals or just below the pubic bone.

Crown and root is usually the final hold in a massage. If your partner is dizzy or feels "spacey," an additional hold involves the feet. Holding their feet draws energy down, relieving the dizziness.

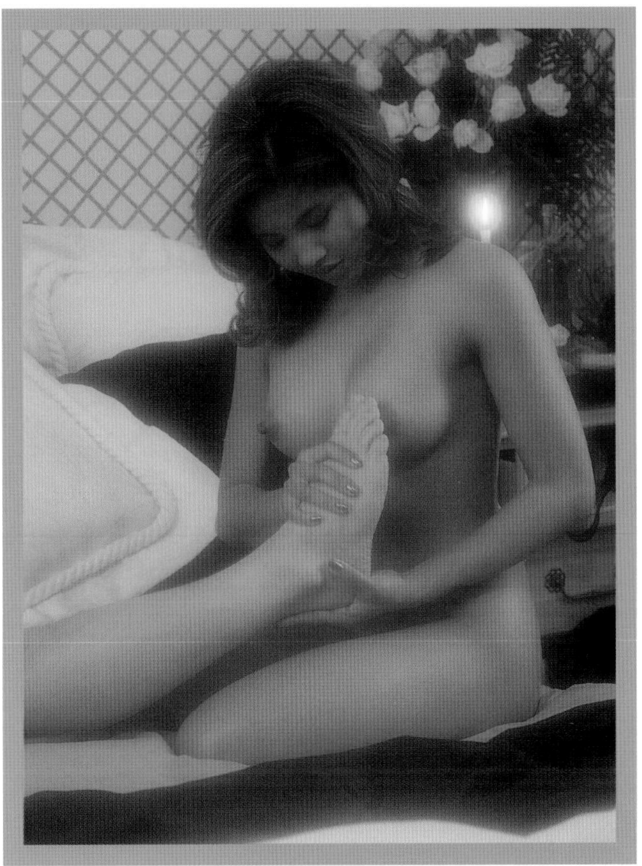

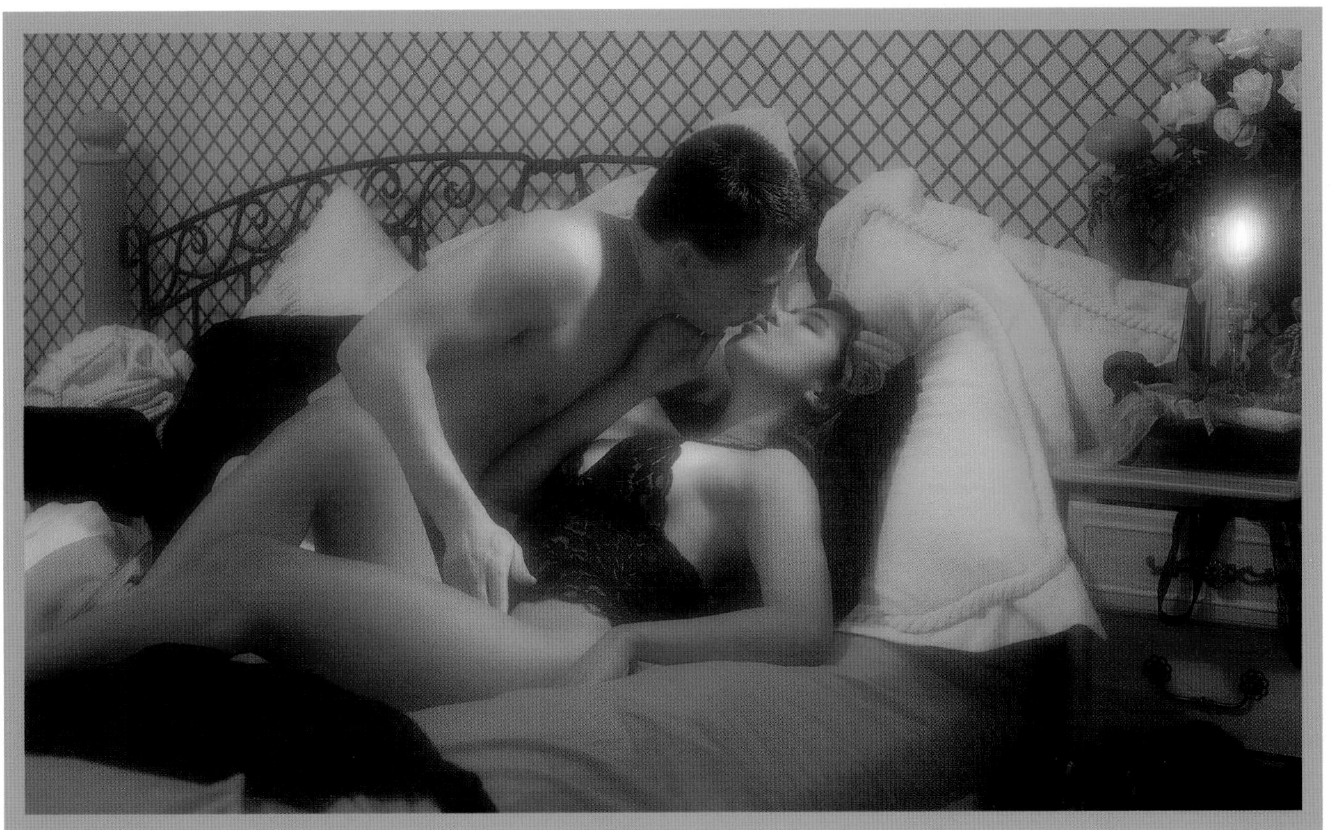

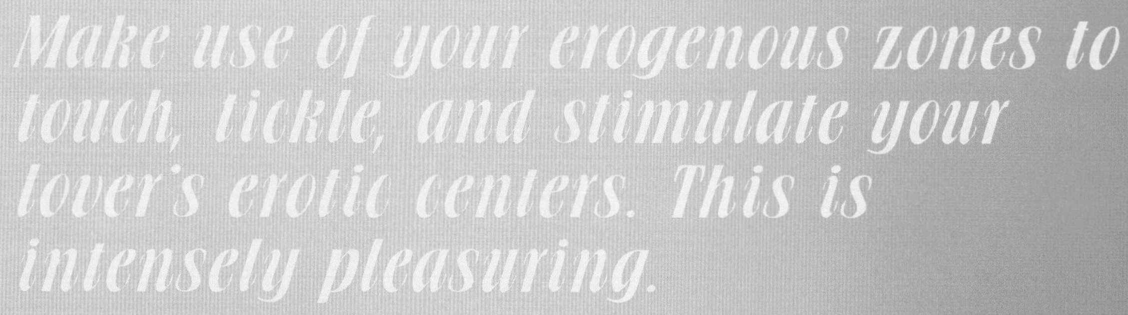
Make use of your erogenous zones to touch, tickle, and stimulate your lover's erotic centers. This is intensely pleasuring.

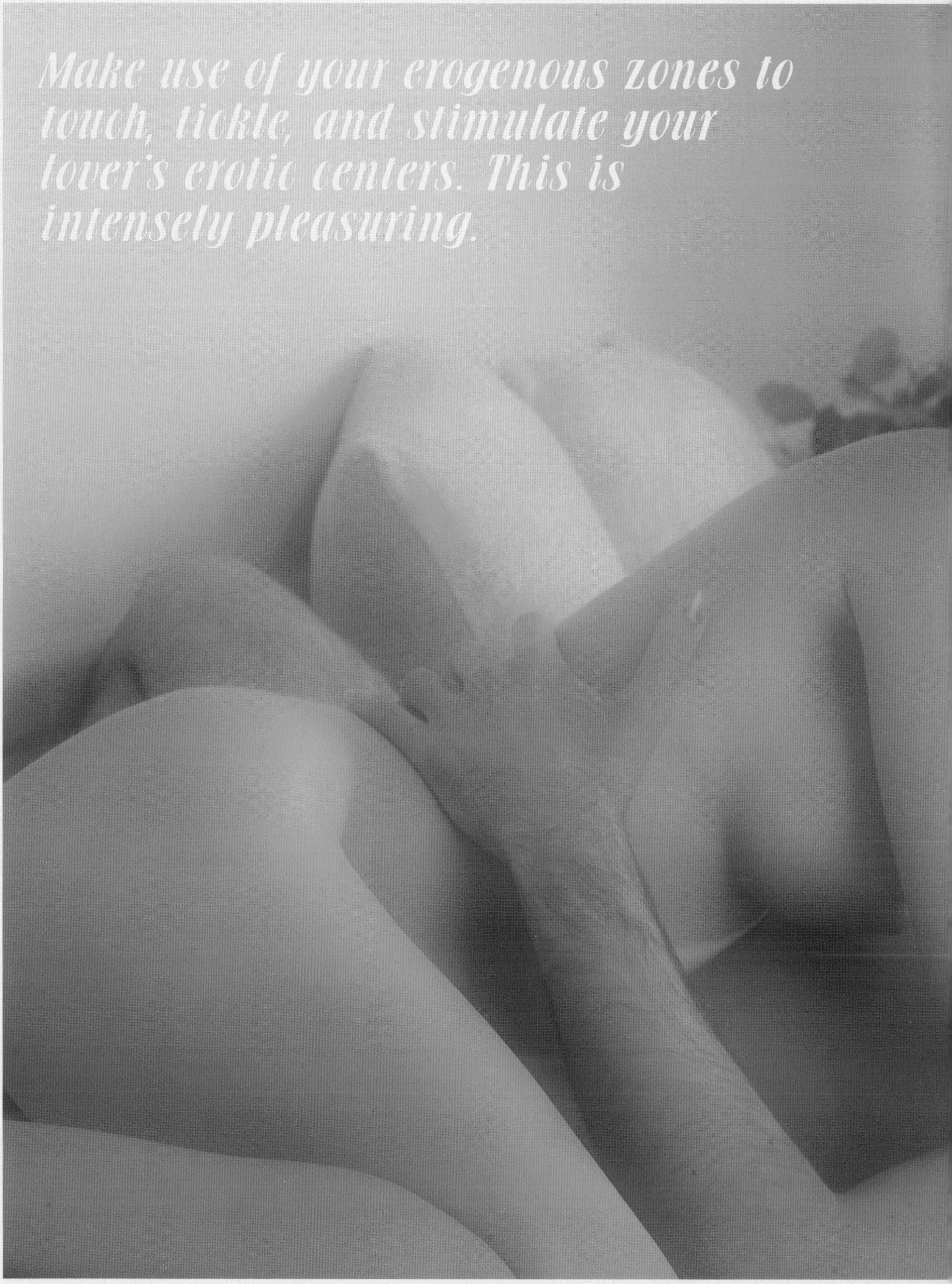

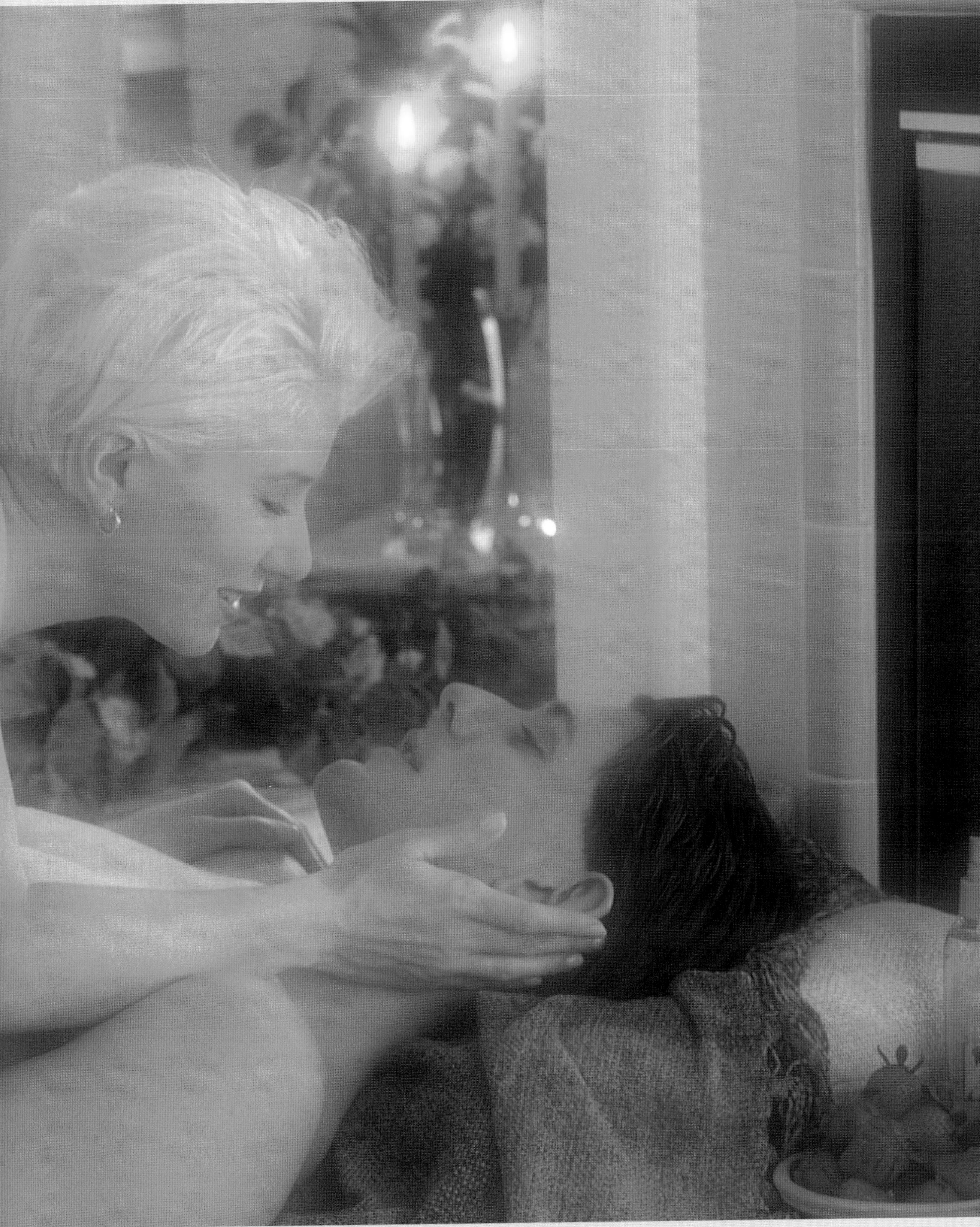

chapter nine

Erogenous Zones

Erogenous zones — those areas of the body that are particularly sensitive to touch and sexual excitation — are focused on throughout a romantic massage, when that is the desired result you wish to achieve.

Obviously, the entire body can be one huge erogenous zone. But there are many individual areas on the body that either have a high concentration of sensory receptors such as: mouth, lips, and fingertips or are highly sensitive because they are rarely touched such as: ears, neck, inner thighs, and nipples.

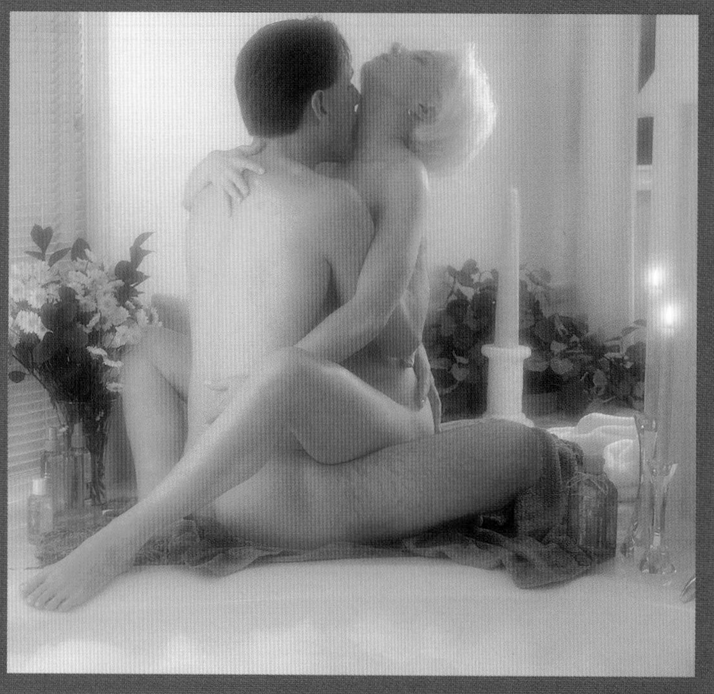

Whatever the reason, there seem to be areas of primary, secondary, and tertiary arousal within these erogenous zones. The trick is to activate each of these sensitized areas in the proper sequence for ultimate sexual arousal. Because each person has different erotic points, you must be aware of your lover's particular needs and desires to realize your mutual goal of pleasuring and satisfaction.

In addition, these techniques for specific sexual arousal should be used as part of your romantic massage. Use your hands to stimulate these erotic areas. Experiment. Use your hair, your eyelashes, your lips, your tongue, your teeth, your chin, your wrists, or your nipples as well as your fingertips. After all, if you utilize your erogenous zones to touch, tantalize, tickle, and stimulate your lover's erogenous zones, imagine the intensity of your sensual pleasuring and satisfaction.

Be creative. Experiment. Remember, time has stopped for the both of you. There is no need to rush any of this. Enjoy your time together.

♥ *"Healthy loving is recognizing that love is never enough. It is being willing to learn the skills that are necessary for nurturing and sustaining an intimate and mutually satisfying relationship.*

♥ *"Healthy loving is aspiring to live in truth and harmony. It is giving freely, receiving graciously, and being thankful, day after day, for the opportunity to be together."*

Jacqui Stratton and Susan Lawton

Secondary Erotic Centers

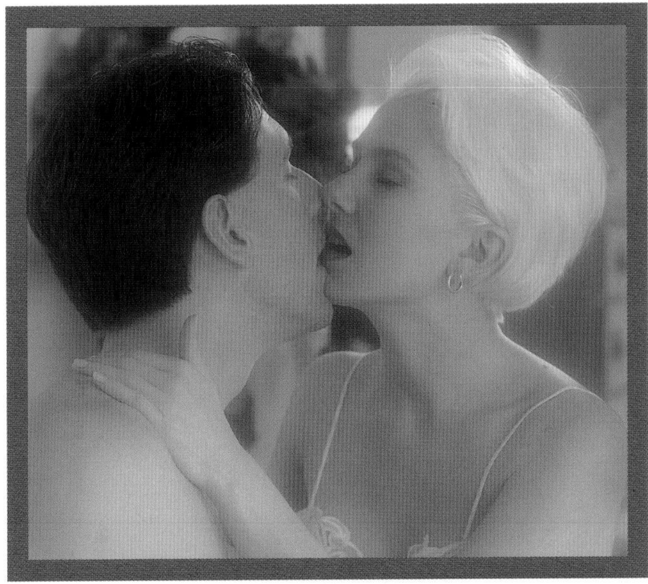

The usual sequence for stimulating erotic pleasure centers is to focus on secondary erogenous zones until sensitized. Then, proceed to primary arousal zones to pique sexual desires. At this point, tertiary areas become highly sensitive to stimulation of any kind.

FACE ♥ The entire face is one erogenous zone. A list of the major zones includes the nose, eyelids, between the eyebrows, the forehead, cheeks, chin, as well as other areas on the head. You may kiss, feather stroke, or lick those areas that are especially sensuous to your lover. If you do not know which areas are most exciting, experiment and ask their opinion of this spot or the next.

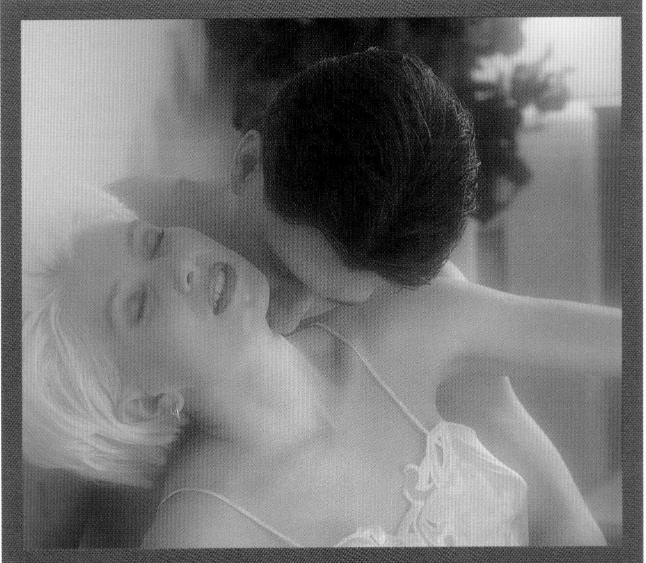

NECK ♥ The front, sides, and back, or nape, of the neck are sensitive, and therefore excitable during massage, nuzzling, and foreplay. Use your lips to lightly drag along the length of the neck between kisses. You will feel the tiny hairs of their neck brush against your lips. Bend back ever so gently and continue on, row by row. Such sensations are at times ticklish, but they are also incredibly stirring.

EARLOBES ♥ Touch each earlobe with your ring finger. The ring finger is somewhat more sensitive to touch than the other fingers, so this will give you pleasure from this experience too. Trace the outline of the ear. Gently massage the earlobe between your thumb and ring finger. The ears can be primary erotic centers for some people, so this massage can trigger "**eargasms.**" Kiss, lick, and delicately nibble each earlobe. Notice your lover's breathing pattern change as they become sexually aroused.

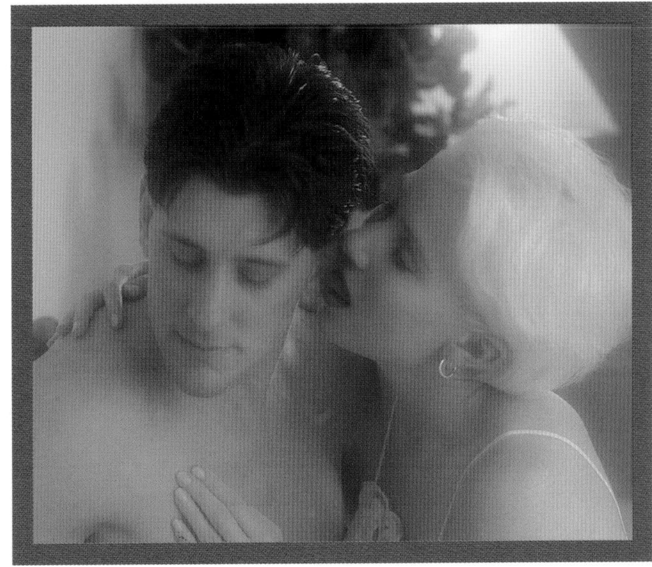

> *"A kiss is something you cannot give without taking and cannot take without giving."*
> *Anonymous*

SHOULDERS & BACK ♥ Caress the shoulders with long light effleurage strokes and kisses as you advance down the length of the spine with soft feathering, using your fingertips and nails. This can send chills and sparks in all directions, because nerves reach out from the spine to every area of the body, transmitting signals of pleasure and pain to the brain for appropriate responses. See if you can raise the responses you are looking for in your lover.

BUTTOCKS & THIGHS ♥ Continue these light feathering strokes down the spine to the sacral triangle — where the triangular-shaped sacrum (base of the spine) meets the gluteal crack of the buttocks — and gently separate the folds of the gluteal cheeks as you brush down the thighs. This area is highly sensitive and, when aroused, is charged with sexual energy. Using your finger nails with ultra light pressure, stroke up between the inner thighs; allow them to part if your lover so chooses. Avoid the anus, perineum, and genitals. Repeat the feathering sequence down the spine and buttocks again.

BEHIND THE KNEES ♥ As you complete the stroking, the kisses, and the blown kisses on the buttocks and thighs, brush lightly behind the knees. Smother this area with lush kisses, licks, and gentle blows of air. If your lover is very ticklish, place your hands on the calf muscles to keep from being kicked in case they involuntarily react to the stimulus of your gentle, teasing licks. Continue feathering the legs down to the soles of their feet, which is another secondary erogenous zone.

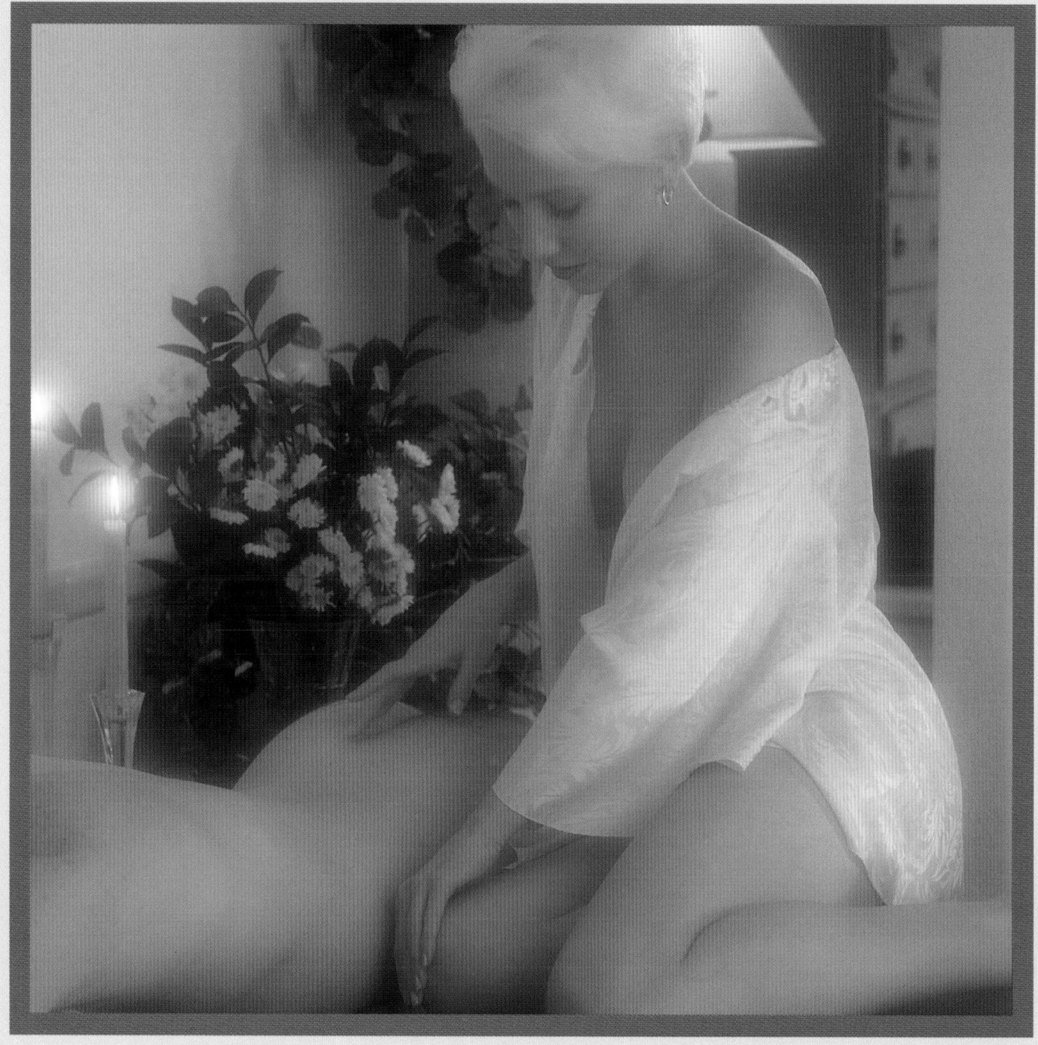

ABDOMEN & NAVEL ♥ Your lover's tummy and navel are other secondary erotic centers. Using the feather stroke in circles around the navel, tease them and tempt them on their abdomen. Draw the circles slower and slower, closer and closer to the navel. As you reach their navel with circles, bend over and tenderly kiss it. Use your hair or possibly a piece of silk or velvet and retrace the circles again. As you finally reach the navel for the second time, kiss and lick the navel with a rotating action.

As you continue your kissing and licking of their navel, spread your kisses and hot breaths in an irregular descending pattern toward your lover's inguinal groove — that area on either side of the genitals that separates the lower abdomen from the upper thighs. You may kiss here and even down to the pubic area, but no further for now.

SIDES & INNER ARMS ♥ While paying your full attention to the lower abdomen, use your hands to gradually caress your lover's sides and inner arms with touches, tickles, and featherings. As you stroke down the inner arms, linger at the wrists to tease and please with your fingertips.

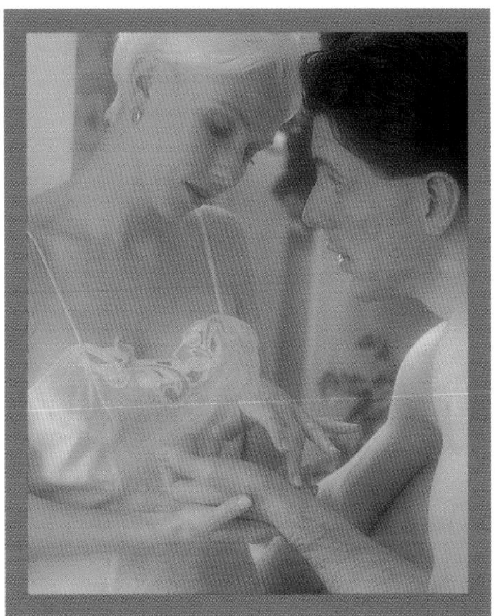

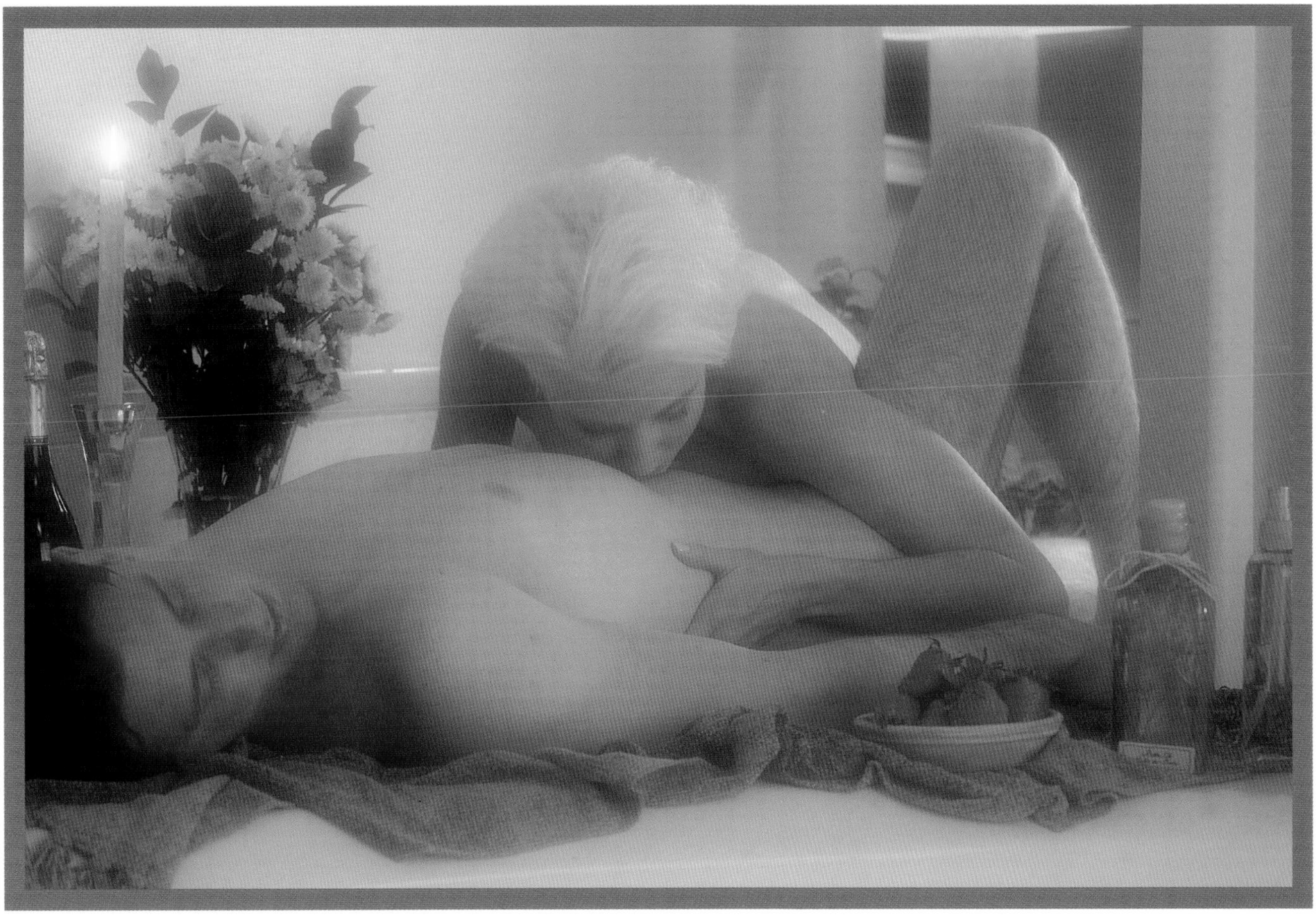

Primary Erotic Centers

LIPS ♥ Your lover's lips are one of the most highly sensitized areas of their body. Because of the large number of nerve receptors on the lips, they are acutely perceptive of contact, moisture, temperature, pressure, and texture. Lips can be kissed, licked, brushed, nibbled, gently pulled, and more.

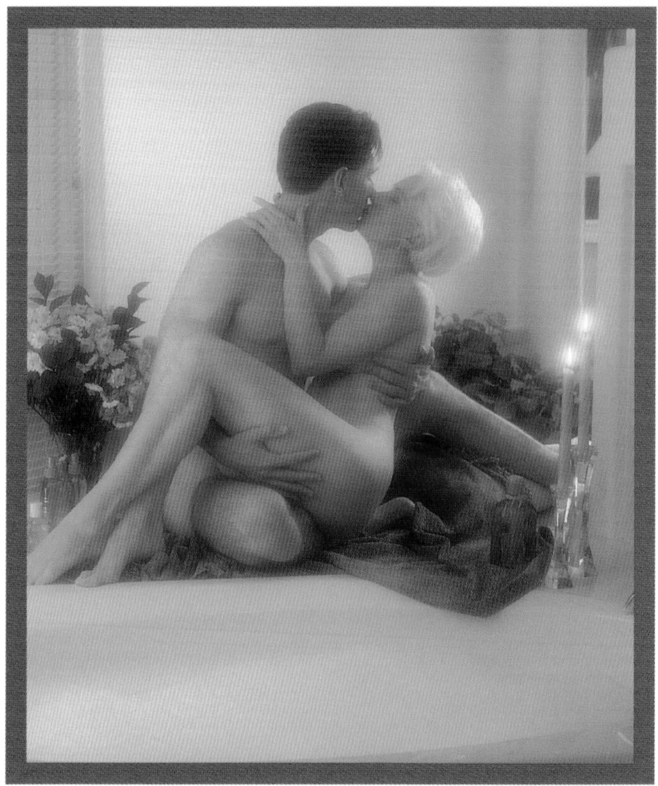

MOUTH & TONGUE ♥ Even though your partner's mouth and tongue do not have as high a concentration of nerve endings as the lips, they are considered major erogenous zones. It is because part of stimulation is not only tactile, but oral also. Use your mouth and tongue to kindle the erotic aspects of romance in your lover's mouth and tongue as you kiss. Make their other erotic zones tingle as they shudder with pleasure.

BREASTS & NIPPLES ♥ Other than lips and genitals, nipples are probably the most erogenous of all the areas of the body. This is true of men and women. Be tender and graceful in your approach to arouse the breast and nipples. Gently pull on them. Twist them slightly. Squeeze them a little. Kiss them, lick them, blow on them. Add edible items like whipped cream, warm fruit preserves, honey or sauces to the breast. Tickle your lover's nipples by batting your eye lashes on them. Massage their breasts using your breasts — an absolutely wild sensation.

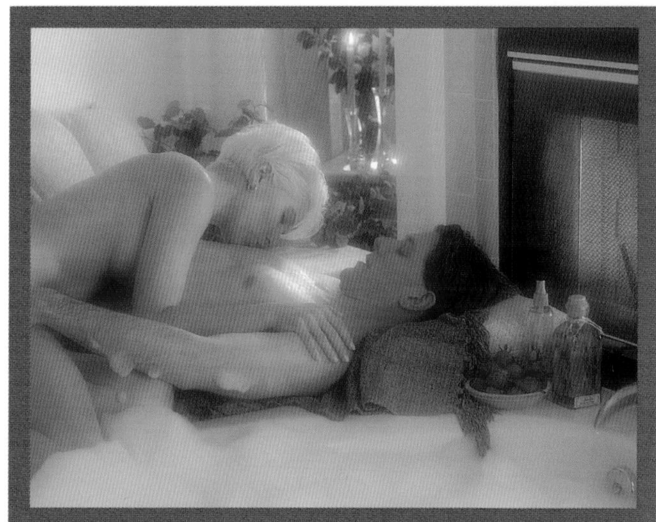

Bath of Desire

4 drops peppermint oil — 10-15 drops magnolia oil — 10 drops orange blossom oil

Place two drops of peppermint oil in an ice cube tray and freeze solid before running bath water.

Run a hot bath, adding magnolia, orange blossom, and remaining peppermint oil to running water. Swirl water until oils are blended. Place ice cubes in a bowl within reach of bathtub.

Climb into full bathtub and soak until warm. Take an ice cube in each hand and rub all over body. Repeat until all ice cubes are melted.

GENITALS ♥ A person's sex, or reproductive, organs are as sensitive, if not more so, as the lips. When they are awakened by being touched, brushed, and caressed, the genitals display an indescribable list of the most highly erotic sensations. All too often, people rush into intimacy, wanting to satisfy or be satisfied quickly. But making love should be savored like sipping the finest brandy, even if intercourse is not the ultimate goal. Explore the genitals and perineum with touches and tickles that are pleasing.

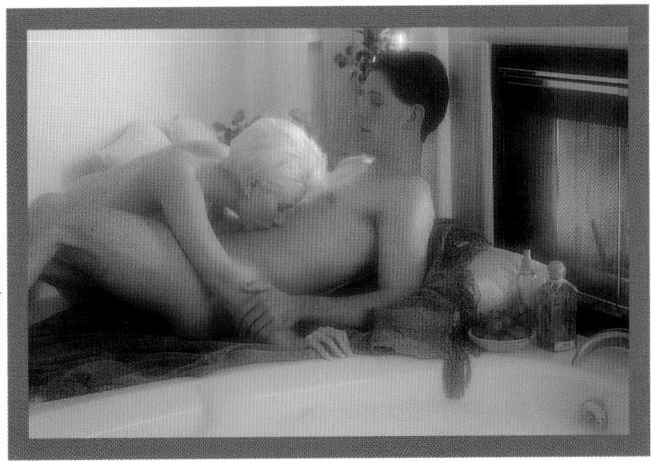

Tertiary Erotic Centers

HANDS & FINGERS ♥ Of all the senses, touch is the most exquisite because it involves the entire body. Touch is also two-way communication in addition to receiving input. Our hands play a crucial role in the sense of touch both to define and shape the world around us, and in touching others' lives. So, it makes sense that our hands and fingers can be a source of sensuous pleasure. The fingertips contain many nerve receptors to record information. By touching lightly, we excite these receptors in ourselves.

As you massage your lover or tease and explore erogenous zones of their body, you cannot help but arouse yourself sexually, because you are using the very erotic areas that excite others — your hands and fingers.

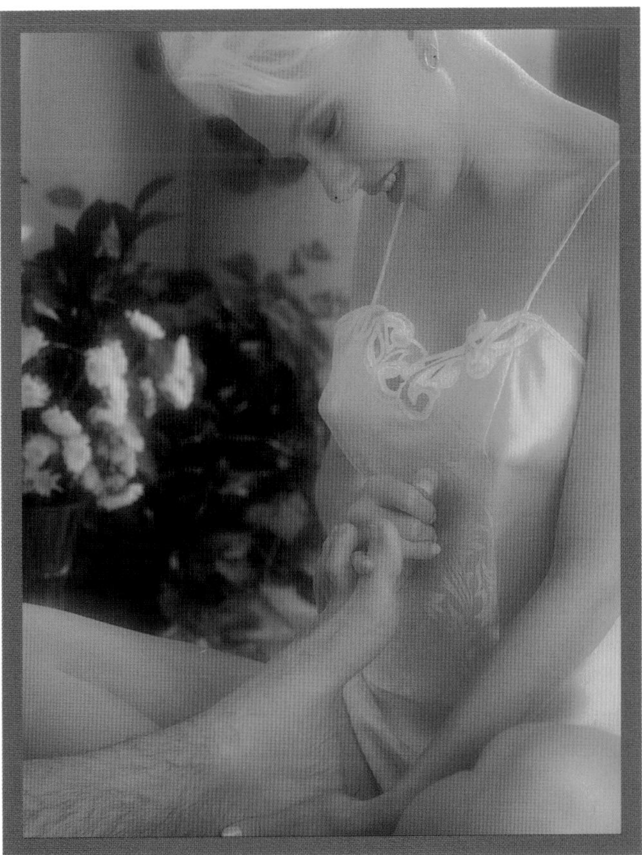

FEET ♥ Among all the areas of the body that people find ticklish, feet are probably the most common. So, when touching or massaging your lover's feet treat them the way your lover likes. Do not move fast or lightly if they are ticklish. Try slow massaging in between the toes, on the ankles, and their arches.

> *"You will sit here, some quiet Summer night, listening to the puffing trains, but you will not be lonely, for these things are a part of me. And my love will go on speaking to you through the chairs, and the tables, and the pictures, as it does now, through my voice, and the quick, necessary touch of my hand."*
>
> *Amy Lowell*

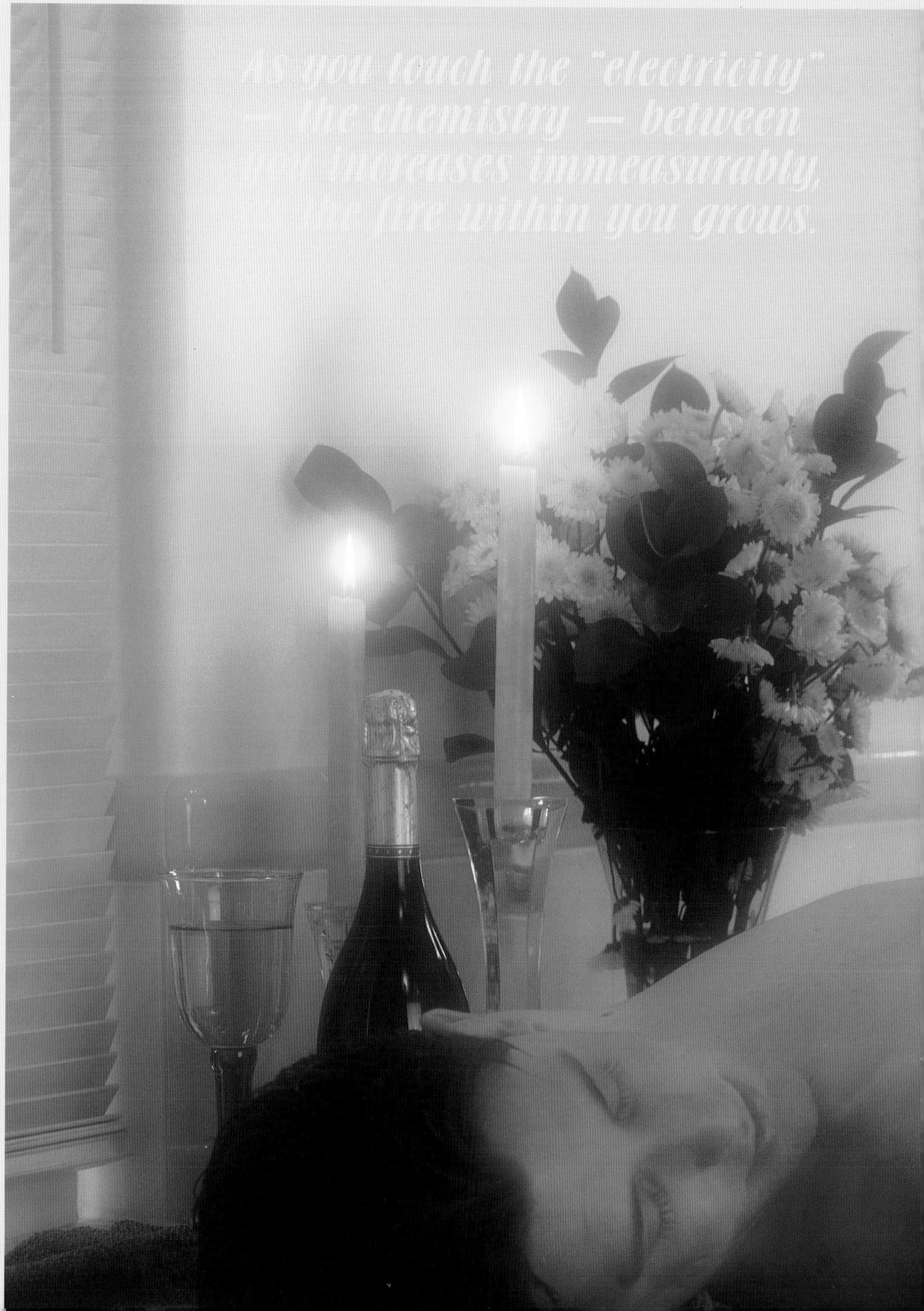

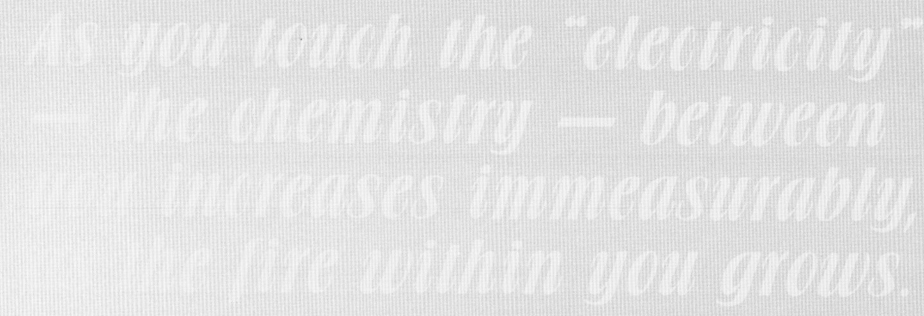
As you touch the "electricity"
— the chemistry — between
increases immeasurably,
fire within you grows.

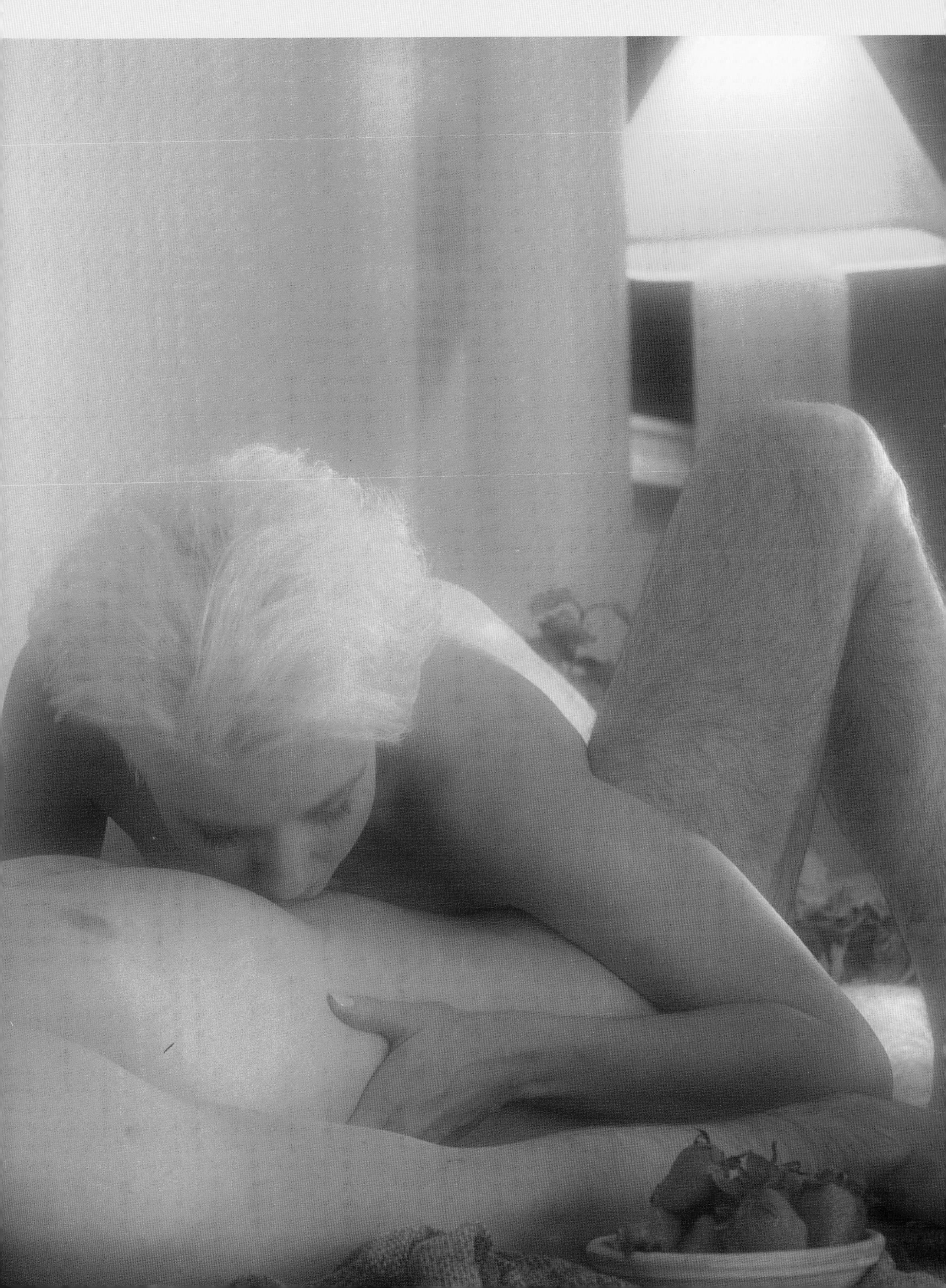

chapter ten

A Prelude...

Regardless of the ultimate goal in romantic massage, enjoy the precious time you share with your lover. In the hectic pace of work and responsibilities, the projects and commitments, the timelines and restraints that we place upon ourselves and have placed by others, we often hope that our loved ones will understand and accept these temporary inconveniences that steal personal moments away. The fact is, we tend to ignore those we hold dear in an attempt to financially provide for them and our future. Isn't it time to enjoy the romance again?

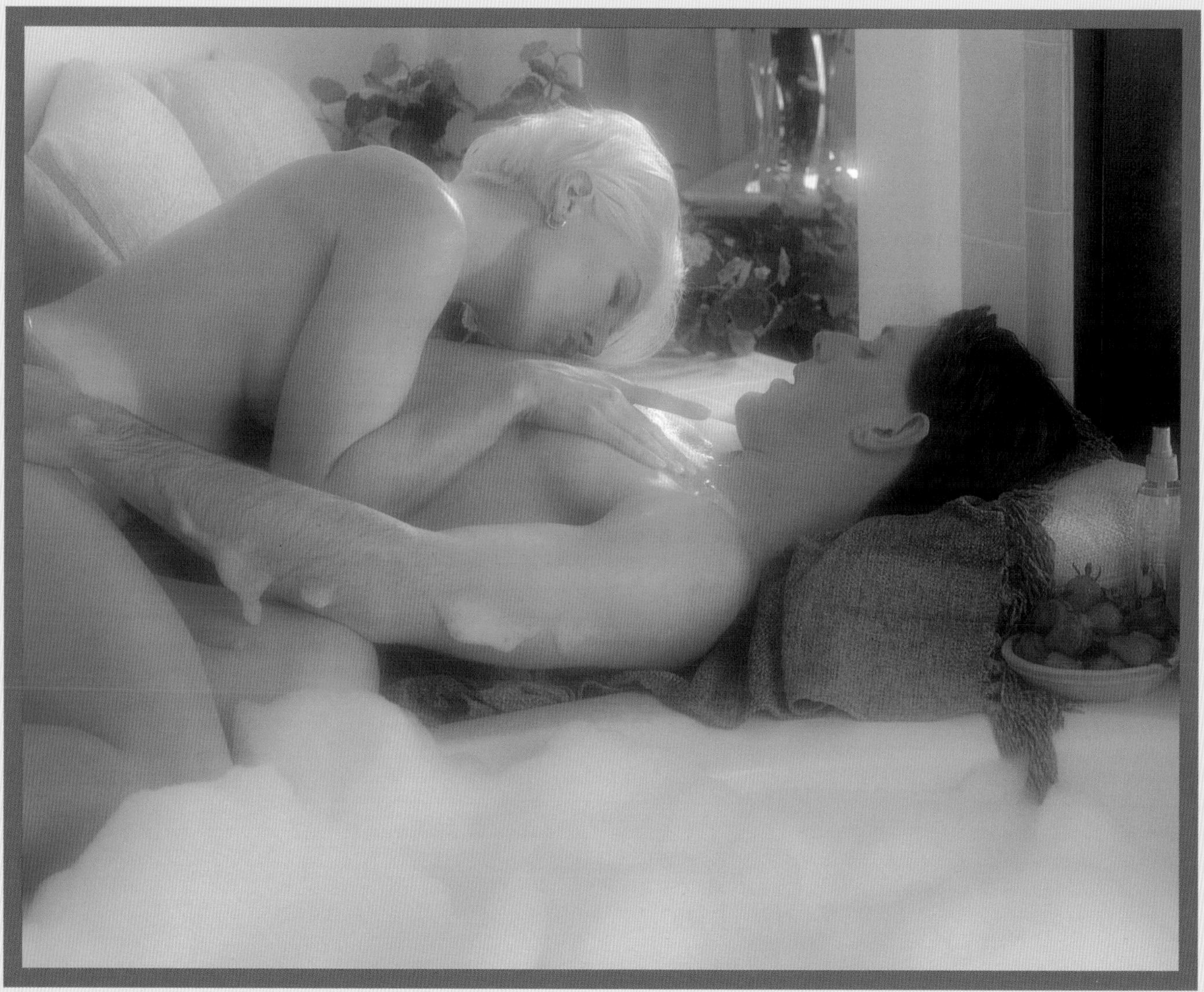

Before this trend of setting your partner and family off to the side adversely affects your personal and intimate relationships, schedule and plan time away from those other distractions and show your lover how much they mean to you.

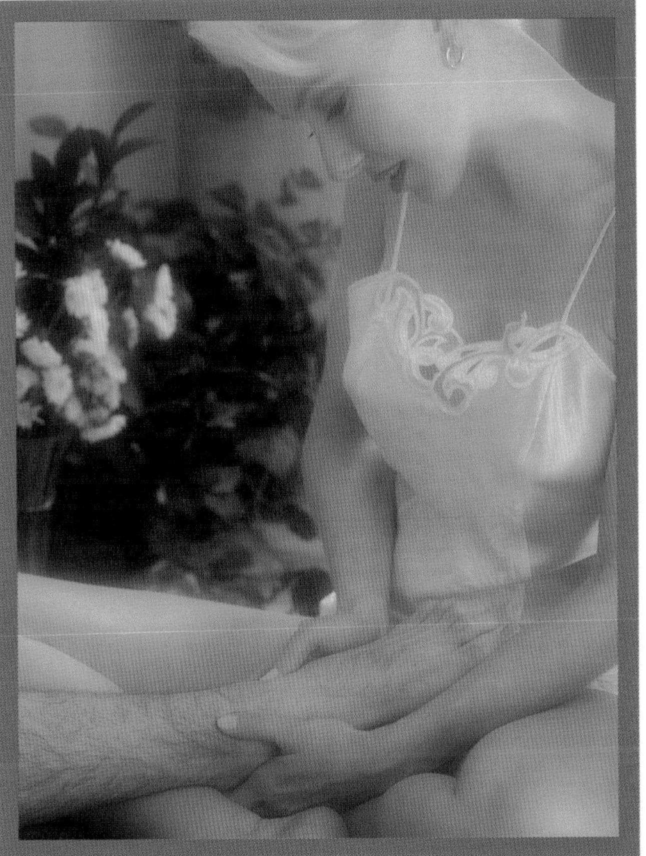

Therapeutic Techniques

After a long day on the go, your partner may greatly appreciate a foot bath in mineral salts and a thorough massage of their feet as described in chapter six. The intent is not so much romance or sex, but to tend to their aches and pains. Show your love in service and nurturing care. The same is the case for a shoulder and back rub as outlined in the beginning of chapter five. This type of massage feels great to someone who carries burdens in their profession or has a physically demanding job.

As your Swedish massage skills help them to relax and ease the pains of the day, your partner may unwind enough to reciprocate the favor. This in itself, could lead to something more intimate later on in the evening or during the weekend.

Therapeutic massage relieves tension and stress and plants the seeds of love and concern that enhance personal relationships later on. Who knows when your loving partner may arrive home one day with airline tickets to an exotic getaway, or a vacation aboard an ocean liner. Even if it's a cozy cabin in the woods or a hiking trip, it's time alone to enhance the romance between you.

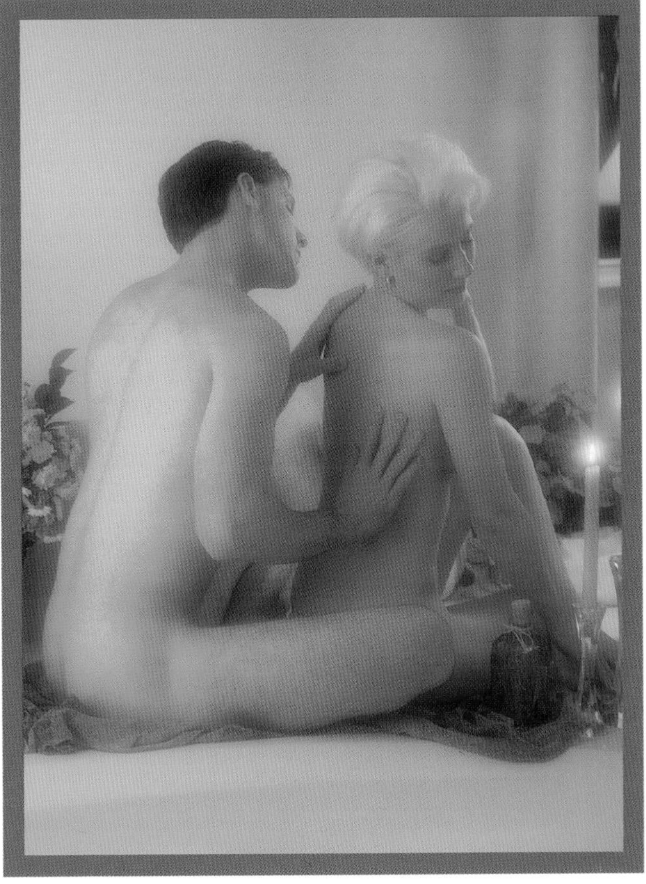

'O, the red rose whispers of passion
And the white rose breathes of love.
O, the red rose is a falcon,
And the white rose is a dove.

But I send you a cream-white rosebud
With a flush on its petal tips,
For the love that is purest and sweetest
Has a kiss of desire on the lips.'

John Boyle O'Reilly

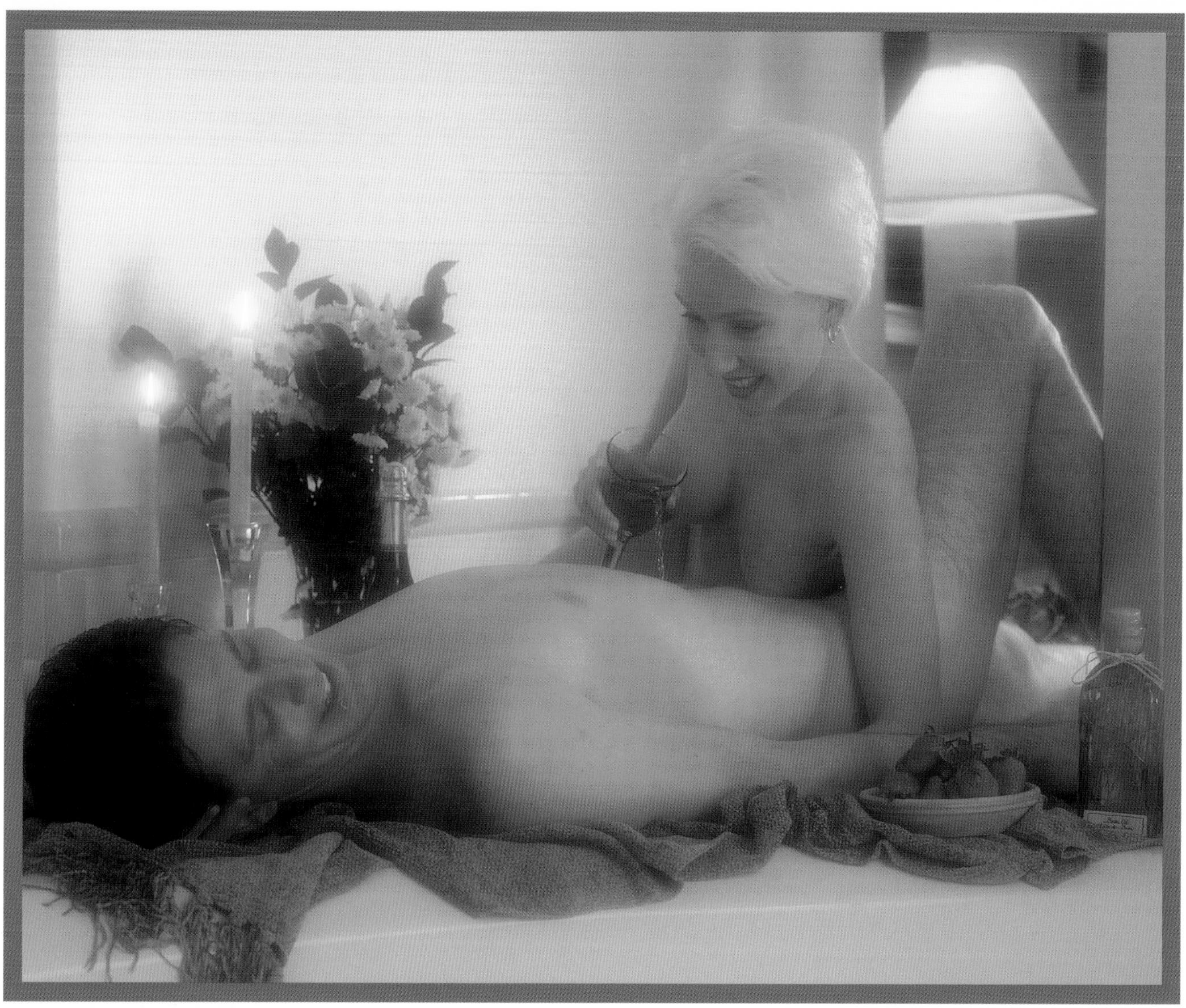

Playful Exploration

If you are searching for something more sensual without necessarily wanting to have intercourse, try sensual massage. Just do not stimulate the erogenous zones.

Situations that may make an erotic or sexual massage unwanted include: impotence/frigidity, depression and loss of libido, menstruation, menopause, advanced stages of pregnancy or recovering from childbirth. During these times, you want to be sensitive to your lover's particular needs. Approach touch with cuddles and hugs, warm blankets or cool breezes (depending on the environment). Non-threatening touch might be welcome in the way of foot or back rubs without innuendos of sex or intimacy, and reassuring hand holds or interlocked arms.

On the other hand, sensual and erotic may be where both of you would like to climax, but not with actual intercourse. Using romantic massage and sensual teasing of erogenous centers often offers enough pleasure and play, innocent exploration, and sensual arousal.

A Prelude to Intimacy

Should you have sex on your minds, you can begin with Swedish massage strokes to relax muscles and relieve mental tension. Follow this with more sensual stroking and kissing of the erogenous centers.

By teasing slowly and steadily during massage time, you both can bring yourselves to a moment of sex initiation that's mutually agreed. This type of romantic massage is a very tender, private, and intimate time as you endeavor to excite and arouse your lover and bring them to a heightened state of awareness.

Once intercourse has been shared, this romantic massage you so carefully planned and executed does not have to end. The hugging, cuddling, nuzzling, and touching can begin anew. With touches come pecks, kisses, licks, and nibbles that are enjoyed again. Begin again to rub and brush, stroke and tease, and before you know it, you have created an exciting interlude between sexual encounters.

When most people roll over exhausted, you and your partner are just beginning to start another round in what could be an afternoon or evening of total delight. This type of massaging and touching need not end in intercourse, but who knows what sparks will fly when two people are so much in love. ♥

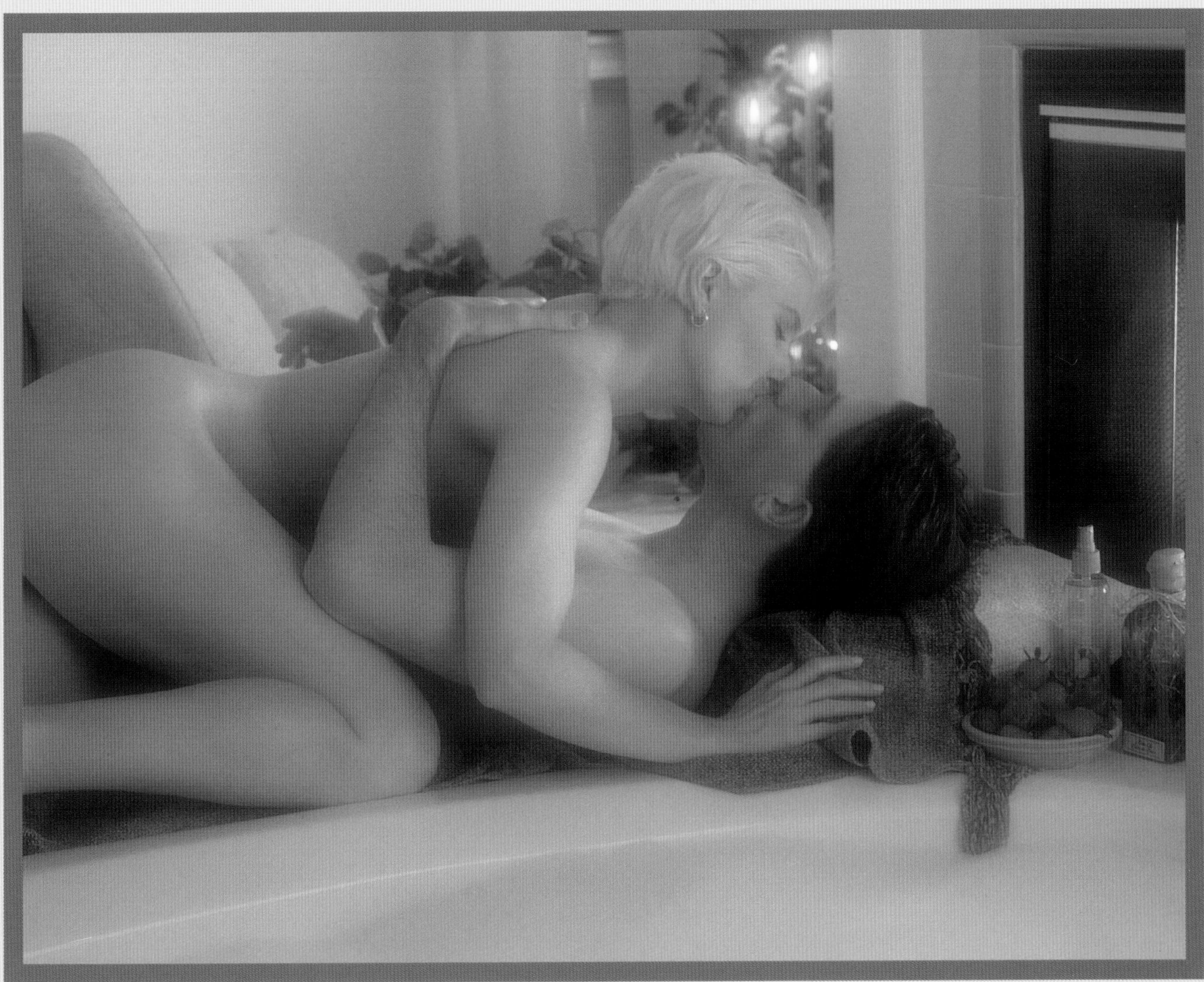

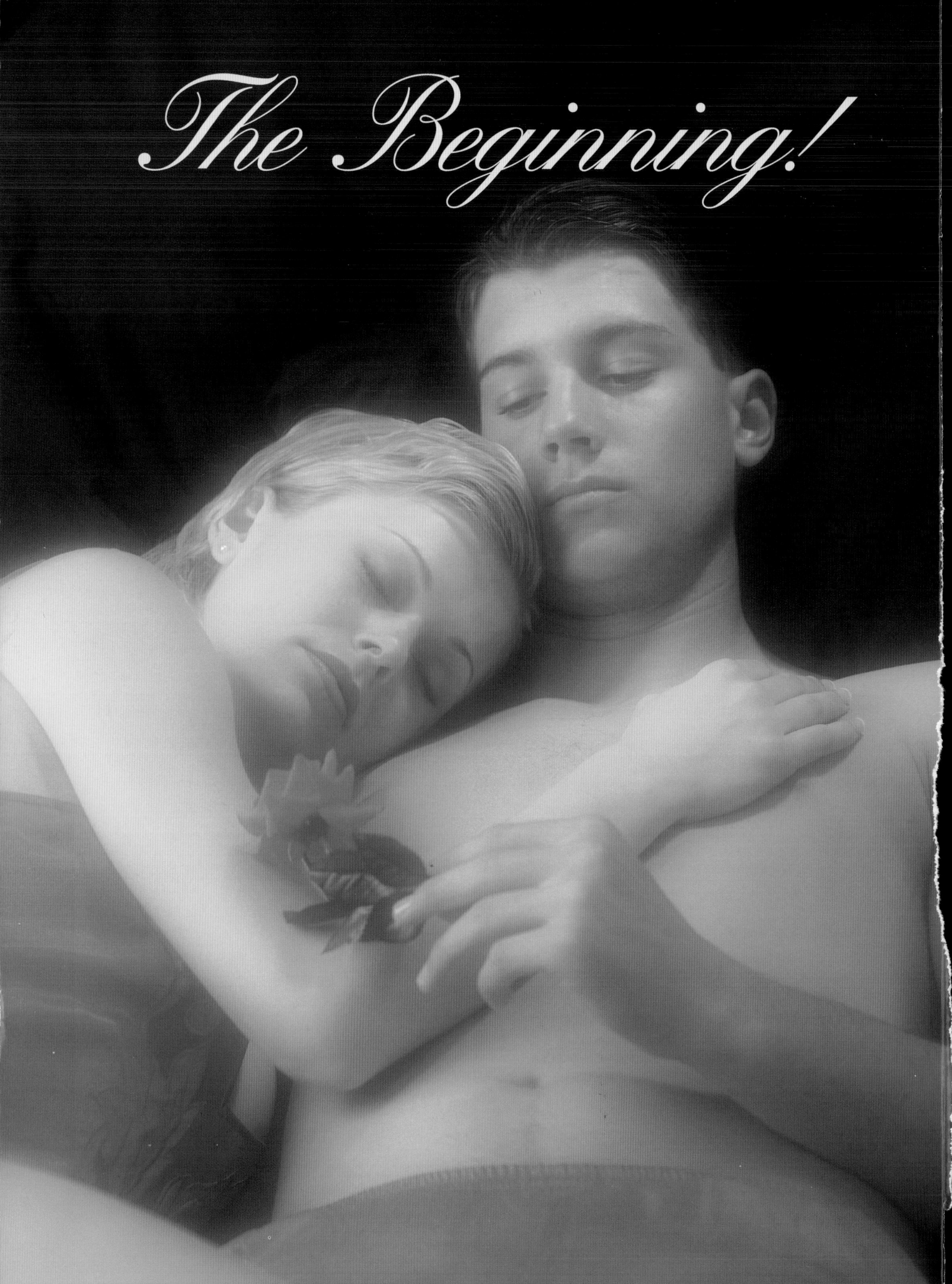
The Beginning!

Index

Metric Conversions

tsp.: teaspoon
tbsp.: tablespoon
8 oz. ounces = 1 cup
32 oz. = 1 quart

¼ tsp.	1.5 milliliters
½ tsp.	2.5 milliliters
1 tsp.	10 milliliters
1 tbsp.	15 milliliters
½ cup	120 milliliters
1 cup	240 milliliters
1 quart	960 milliliters
1 oz.	28 grams